Building Your Future

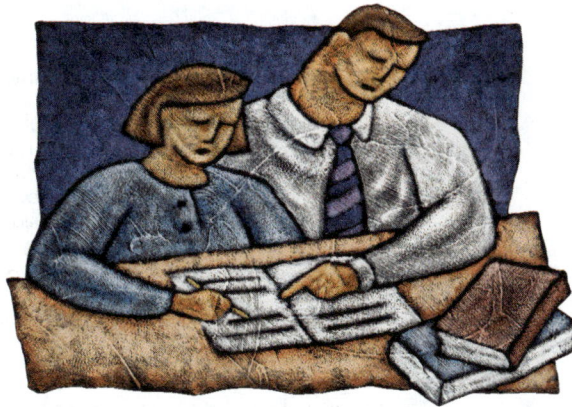

Sally R. Campbell
Consumer Economics Author and Consultant
Winnetka, Illinois

Publisher
The Goodheart-Willcox Company, Inc.
Tinley Park, Illinois

Library of Congress Cataloging-in-Publication Data

Campbell, Sally R.
Building your future / Sally R. Campbell. -- 2nd ed.
        p. cm. -- (Transitions)
Includes index.
ISBN 978-1-60525-129-5
        1. Teenage pregnancy. 2. Teenage mothers. 3. Parenting. 4. Teenagers--
Sexual behavior. I. Title.
RG556.5.C35 2009
618.200835--dc22

                                                                    2009011517

About the Author

Sally R. Campbell is a freelance writer and consultant in consumer economics and personal finance. She develops educational materials, including textbooks, teacher guides, curriculum guides, and student activity materials. Sally maintains an interest in young consumers and has researched the financial and employment aspects of teen parenting.

Formerly, Sally was the editor and assistant director of the Money Management Institute of Household International, a provider of consumer loans and credit. There she wrote educational materials related to money management and financial planning.

Sally holds a master's degree in education from St. Louis University and completed the Certified Financial Planning Professional Education Program of the College for Financial Planning. She taught Family and Consumer Sciences as well as consumer education in St. Louis schools.

Acknowledgments

We would like to thank the following professionals who reviewed the original text and provided valuable input:

Cathy Allison
GRADS Coordinator
Auburn Career Center
Concord, Ohio

Dawn Gale Aspacher
Parent Educator
Child and Family Resources, Inc.
The Center for
Adolescent Parents
Tucson, Arizona

JoAnn J. Bartek
FCS Teacher/Director, Student Parent
Team SCLC
Lincoln High School
Lincoln, Nebraska

Martha Hamdani-Swain
former Program Coordinator,
Pregnancy Education and Parenting
Program
Jack Yates High School
Houston, Texas

Sheree M. Moser
FCS Department Chair
and District Assistant
Lincoln High School
Lincoln, Nebraska

Sara McDonald Rohar
Project Director, Young Mother's
Program
Birmingham City Schools
Birmingham, Alabama

Table of Contents

Introduction

Today the future may seem like it's a long way off. With all you have to do and decide right now, it might seem like decisions about the future can wait. Actually, however, the choices you make and the actions you take now will help set your future course.

As a parent, you have many new responsibilities, decisions, and matters to manage for yourself and your child. These tasks may seem complicated, but they're crucial to your family's well-being.

Building Your Future was written to help you understand these new responsibilities. It covers many topics, including the following:

- ☞ understanding legal matters
- ☞ managing money and resources
- ☞ being a wise shopper
- ☞ handling credit, insurance, and financial accounts
- ☞ setting goals for your education, training, and career
- ☞ preparing for the workforce and finding a job
- ☞ balancing your many roles

Much of the language in this book is directed to young mothers, but, a young father can gain just as much by reading this book. His support and involvement are just as valuable as the mother's. Even if you and your baby's other parent are not together, each of you still has much to offer your child.

Your baby may be a girl or a boy. To make the chapters easier to read, we have referred to your baby in some sections as he and in other sections as she. We hope this will also help you relate to the chapters in a personal way as you think about your child. Do all you can to prepare the best possible future for yourself and your child!

Chapter 1
Getting the
Help You Need

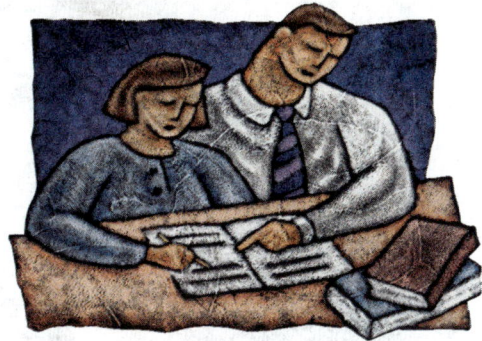

Being a pregnant or parenting teen can be very demanding at times. You may feel overwhelmed by all there is to do and decide. You might even feel lonely, but it can be comforting to know you are not alone. There are many sources of help available. You just have to know where to look.

This chapter will help you think about what kinds of help you might need. You will learn where to look for this assistance. This chapter will also give you tips for seeking help and dealing with social service agencies.

What Kind of Help Do You Need?

Before you start your search, think about the support you already have. Will your partner stand by your side? Will your family and his family be supportive? Are there others you can count on in difficult times? Being able to rely on help from friends and family members can make things easier for you, but if this isn't an option, there are many other sources of support.

It may help to talk with a trusted adult about your situation. This might be a parent, relative, or friend's mother. A guidance counselor or teacher could also help. A trusted adult can listen to your concerns and advise you about the choices you will need to make over the next few months. See Figure 1-1. Finding a good listener is important, too.

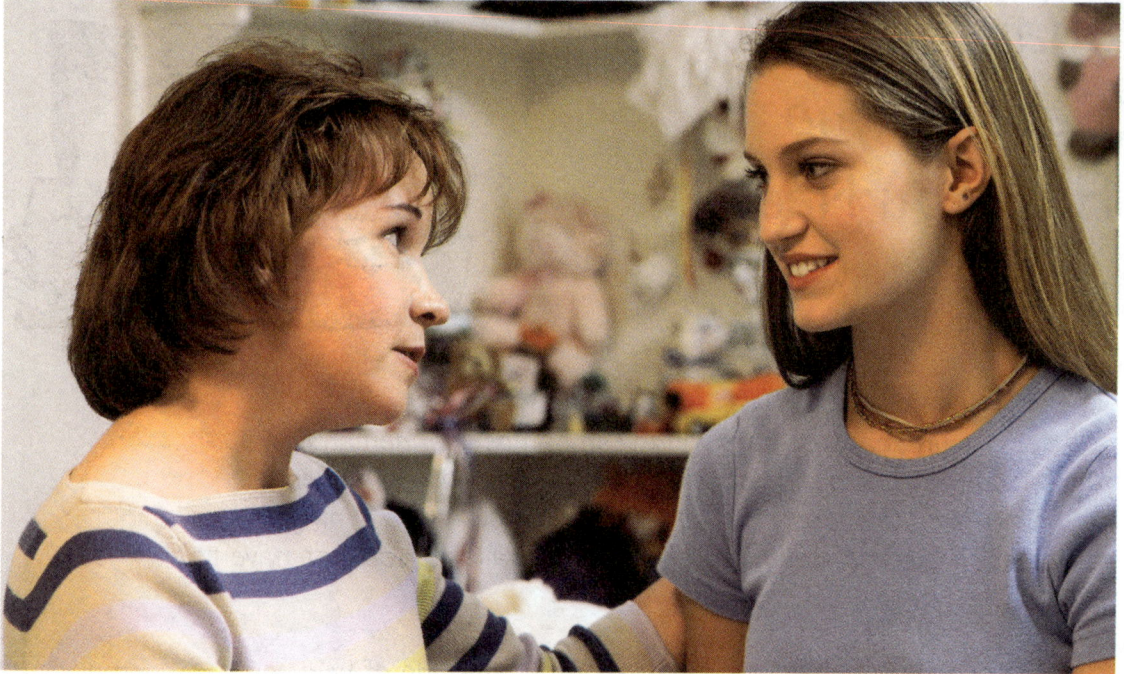

1-1 Talking with a trusted adult can help you make many of the important decisions you face.

Your next task is to decide what kinds of help you think you'll need most. Each situation is unique. Your specific needs may differ from those of another pregnant teen. Many pregnant teens share some of the following basic needs:

- emotional support
- information on options related to pregnancy
- guidance with decision making
- financial assistance
- assistance with medical care, food, or housing
- programs for continuing education and job training

Places to Look for Help

Once you have decided what help you need, it's time to start your search. It's best to start as early as you can. This gives you the most time possible to find out what kinds of help are available. The following sections describe common places you can turn for assistance.

Telephone Hot Lines

You may feel uneasy talking to people you know. If so, calling a crisis hot line might be an option. This can give you someone to talk with who may be able to help. You can find hot line numbers in the Yellow Pages of your phone book under <u>Crisis</u>, <u>Pregnancy</u>, or <u>Hospitals and Clinics</u>. You may find others listed under <u>Youth Services</u> or <u>Social Service Agencies</u>. In the White Pages, you might also look for a listing of <u>Crisis Pregnancy Center</u> or <u>Planned Parenthood</u>.

Many hot lines can give you information and referrals. A referral is a suggestion of a place to go for specific services you may need. A referral may include

- ☛ agency's name, address, and phone number
- ☛ a brief description of the agency's services
- ☛ the name of a contact person at the agency

The people who answer hot lines calls are trained to listen and offer support. Often they can give sound advice. The person who answers your call should be caring, open-minded, and eager to help you. Just talking through your concerns with someone who cares can be a great comfort.

Internet Sources

The Internet is a vast network of resources you can use to visit sites on the World Wide Web. These Web sites have information about countless topics and organizations. You can use the Web to learn more about pregnancy and related issues. Some Web sites just offer basic information. Others describe specific types of help that are available to you.

To use the Internet, you will need a computer with Internet access and a browser. A browser is a tool that helps guide you through Web sites. Two common browsers are Microsoft Internet Explorer and Netscape Navigator.

If you don't have a computer or Internet access at home, visit your public or school library. Most libraries have at least one computer where you can go online. If you need help, ask a librarian to show you how to use the Internet. You may also be able to use your school's computer lab.

To find information online, you may want to use a search engine. This is a tool that searches the World Wide Web for specific information. Each search engine has a Web site through which you can access it. Once you're on the Web site for the search engine, enter a key word to help you find the information you seek. Be as specific as possible. The search engine will give you a list of matches for your key word. From this list, choose any Web sites that interest you. By clicking on a listed site, the computer will take you right to that site.

You can use the Internet to find the information you need. Be cautious, though. Not all the information you will find is reliable. Some of it is even untrue. Depend mostly on reputable sites. These include sites run by the government, professional agencies, and well-known companies. You can also look at the date on the site. When was it created or last updated? Is the information current? If you're unsure about information you find, do some research to verify the facts.

Government Agencies

City, county, state, and federal governments each provide a variety of services. A good place to find an overview of these services may be the government section in your local phone book. This section is also sometimes called the Blue Pages. If your phone book does not have these listings, look for more information at your public library. Each state also has its own government Web site, which you can access to learn more.

Department of Health and Human Services

The U.S. Department of Health and Human Services is an office that focuses on meeting the health and service needs of the public. This federal department offers a broad range of programs that are supported by federal tax dollars.

Many of the agencies and programs of this department are listed in the government section of the phone book. You can also learn more at your library or the Web site for this department. The U.S. Department of Health and Human Services has information and referrals on a number of topics. See Figure 1-2. You may find some of these services helpful.

Many states also have a department of health and human services. Not all of these departments go by this same name. Contact your state's department to learn more about its programs.

Department of Health and Human Services Programs

The Department of Health and Human Services operates many programs that might assist you. From these programs, you can get information or referrals on the following topics:

- adoption
- AIDS prevention and treatment
- alcoholism or drug abuse prevention and treatment
- child abuse
- child care
- child support
- domestic violence prevention and services
- education
- employment services or job training
- financial aid
- family planning
- food programs
- health care
- health insurance
- immunizations
- Medicaid
- mental health care
- nutrition
- parenting education
- prenatal care
- sexually transmitted disease prevention and treatment
- TANF program
- WIC Bureau

1-2 The U.S. Department of Health and Human Services offers help and programs in a wide variety of areas.

The U.S. Department of Health and Human Services funds public aid programs. The primary financial aid program is the Temporary Assistance for Needy Families (TANF) Bureau. This program replaces the former program, Aid to Families with Dependent Children (AFDC).

States receive grants from the federal government to run their TANF Bureaus. Each state decides who is eligible to receive aid. States also decide what benefits and services they will offer. All states have school and work requirements. They also impose lifetime limits on receiving aid. In most cases, pregnant or parenting teens are required to live with their parents in order to qualify for benefits. Some allow you to receive benefits as long as you're a full-time student. Contact your public aid office to learn about the TANF Bureau in your state.

The federal and state departments of health and human services work together to run the Medicaid program. This program pays health care costs for needy individuals and families. If you qualify for the TANF Bureau, you will likely also qualify for Medicaid. You may qualify for Medicaid even if you don't qualify for TANF.

You may also qualify for help under the Special Supplemental Nutrition Program for Women, Infants, and Children (WIC). This program is also run by the government. It serves women who are pregnant or breast-feeding, as well as their infants and young children. WIC clients may qualify to receive some or all of the following services:

- ☞ food benefits. These benefits come in the form of vouchers that are like coupons. They can be used at grocery stores to pick up the items listed at no cost. Foods often covered are infant formula, milk, cereal, juice, peanut butter, eggs, beans, and rice. Receiving these food items can help parents stretch their money farther. Some programs are now using plastic cards that look like credit cards instead of vouchers.
- ☞ nutrition information and counseling. Dietitians can teach parents about foods and nutrition. They can help them learn to provide more healthful meals for their families.

☞ medical screening and referrals. Some programs have nurses
on their staff who do health screenings. These nurses may
track a child's health and growth. They might follow the
progress of a woman's pregnancy. The nurses can also refer
clients to the medical services they need.

To qualify for WIC, you must meet income guidelines. You must
also be pregnant, breast-feeding, or the parent of a young child. To
find out more, contact your public aid office or health department.
These offices can refer you to the nearest WIC office.

The States Children's Health Insurance Program (SCHIP) is a
national program that helps insure children who are not insured.
This program gives each state money to provide insurance. Your
public aid office can tell you more about this program. Ask what
your state offers under this program and whether your baby can
receive this coverage.

Your baby needs to have immunizations to protect his health. If
you cannot afford these, your child may be able to get them free
through the Vaccines for Children Program (VFC). Ask your local
health department what the requirements are for this program.

Department of Education

Your local school district is a government office. It is a part of
your state department of education. Your school district runs the
public schools in your area. It decides what programs each school
will have and what funds each program will receive. The district also
funds any special programs for pregnant and parenting teens. It
may also pay for child care provided by the school, too. Ask your
teachers or counselor what programs are offered in your district.
Then you can choose whether to participate in these programs.

If you need public aid, you must meet many requirements. One
is you must stay in school. If you're 16 years or older, you may be
able to meet this requirement by participating in the General
Educational Development program. This program lets you earn a
general equivalency diploma (GED). You could earn this diploma
by taking an exam. You would attend classes to help you

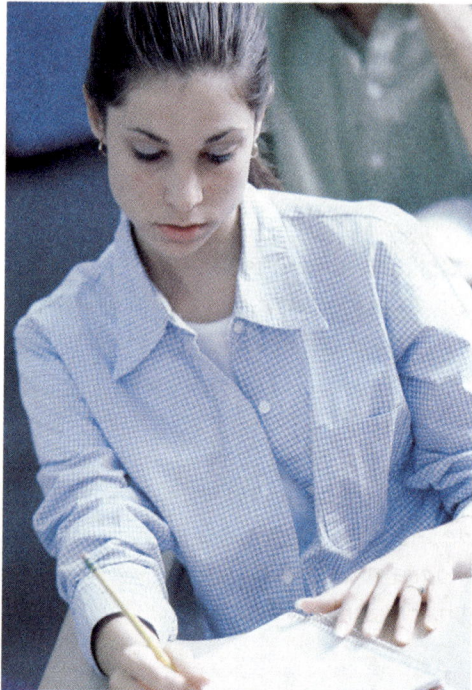

1-3 Preparing for the GED exam takes effort. To pass this test, you'll need to attend classes and study your materials at home.

review for the exam. See Figure 1-3. Passing this exam would mean you have the same basic knowledge as most teens who graduate from high school. Many employers, the military, and most colleges will accept the GED instead of a high school diploma. Ask your school district office if you want to learn more about preparing for the GED.

Department of Housing

Your state or local department of housing may be another source of assistance. This office can help you find and pay for a place to live. Ask your public aid office to help you contact the department of housing. This department can tell you about low-income housing options in your area. A second option may be subsidized housing. This means the government pays part of the rent and you pay the rest. This program is often called Section 8. As with other government programs, you must qualify in order to participate. In some states, age restrictions may apply. This is often 18 years or older.

Social Service Programs

You may also be able to find help through social service programs that are not operated by the government. These programs may operate on a national, state, or local level. Many are unique to your community. Most social service programs are nonprofit agencies, which means they don't operate to make money. Instead, their mission is public service. They offer their help at little or no cost to you. Grants and donations fund these programs.

Figure 1-4 lists examples of social service programs. You can find programs such as these listed in the Yellow Pages of your phone book. You can also ask your counselor, caseworker, or health care provider to refer you to these programs.

Examples of Social Service Agencies

- ❖ Big Brothers/Big Sisters
- ❖ Boys' and Girls' Clubs
- ❖ Catholic Charities
- ❖ child care resource and referral networks
- ❖ community centers
- ❖ counseling services
- ❖ crisis hot lines
- ❖ domestic violence shelters
- ❖ employment and job services
- ❖ family service centers
- ❖ food depositories
- ❖ Habitat for Humanity
- ❖ homeless shelters
- ❖ legal aid services
- ❖ literacy classes
- ❖ parent education agencies
- ❖ parenting hot lines
- ❖ parent networks and services
- ❖ Red Cross
- ❖ Salvation Army
- ❖ special needs services
- ❖ substance abuse treatment centers
- ❖ support groups
- ❖ transitional living centers
- ❖ Travelers' and Immigrants' Aid Society
- ❖ United Charities
- ❖ United Way
- ❖ Urban League
- ❖ YMCA/YWCA
- ❖ youth centers

1-4 You are likely to find these types of social service agencies and programs listed in the Yellow Pages under *Social Service Organizations.*

Religious Organizations

If you belong to a religious group, this may be a good source of help. The members of your group can offer you support and friendship. Some members may know of local services you could use. Others might also be able to help you with child care, housing, food, baby items, and maternity and baby clothes. The members of your house of worship may have much to offer you.

Many houses of worship also offer support programs for single parents. These might include child care centers, parenting classes, and limited health care programs. Your religious leaders may be able to counsel you. They can also refer you to other services you need. In some cases, houses of worship have special funds they use to assist members in need.

Clinics, Hospitals, and Medical Groups

Health care is always important. When you're pregnant or have a child, it matters even more. Find the best medical care you can. You and your baby deserve it. You may need help in the following three areas:

☛ knowing what care is available to you
☛ finding a health care provider
☛ paying for medical care

First, you may wonder what type of care is available to you. Suppose you're covered by your parents' health insurance. Find out whether their policy will cover you during your pregnancy and delivery. Will it cover you after the baby is born? Will it cover your baby? Some companies will provide these kinds of coverage while others do not.

The baby's father might be able to provide health insurance for the baby through his job. If you're not married, he probably won't be able to include you on his policy. He might be able to help pay your medical expenses, though. This would take some of the burden from you.

If you have trouble finding medical care, talk to your counselor or caseworker. This person may be able to refer you to a good provider. Some health care facilities are listed in the government section of the phone book. Others are in the Yellow Pages. You might find them under <u>Obstetrics and Gynecology (OB/GYN)</u> and <u>Pediatric Care</u>. (To learn more about medical care in pregnancy, see another title in this series, <u>Your New Baby</u>.)

If money is a problem, look for low- or no-cost care through a community clinic or county hospital. Your local health department may be able to provide low-cost care. Find out if you qualify for Medicaid through your public aid office. If so, Medicaid will help you and your baby get the medical care you need.

Questions to Ask About Health Care

It's never too soon to look for the health care you and your baby will need. It may not seem clear where to start your search, though. First, decide what type (or types) of provider you need. See Figure 1-5 for types of health care providers. Before you settle on a health care provider, you will want to learn about his or her qualifications. You can use the questions listed in Figure 1-6 to help you rate various health care providers.

You will also want to learn more about the available health care facilities before you go for care. Your options include clinics, hospitals, and health care practices. Don't be afraid to ask questions. Find out the following about any health care facility you're considering:

- ☛ Whom does this facility serve? (Find out if you can receive care at this facility. Will the facility accept your insurance or Medicaid card? If you don't have insurance or Medicaid, can you still receive care?)
- ☛ What services are offered? (Find out if the care you need is available.)
- ☛ Who provides the services? (Look for a provider who is experienced and certified in the field of care you need.)
- ☛ What must you do to receive services? (Find out where to apply, what documents to bring, and what requirements you must meet.)
- ☛ What will services cost and what payment arrangements can you make?
- ☛ What problems might you have in receiving care through this facility?

Types of Health Care Providers

Title	Areas of Care
Physician	a doctor of medicine (MD) or doctor of osteopathy (DO) who is trained and qualified to provide complete medical care; often called a family doctor or general practitioner
Specialist	a physician who completed additional training and education in a specialty such as heart disease, surgery, cancer, pediatrics, or other area of treatment
Gynecologist	a physician who specializes in caring for women's reproductive systems
Obstetrician	a physician who specialized in caring for women during pregnancy and childbirth
Pediatrician	a physician who treats infants and children
Certified Nurse-Midwife	a nurse with advanced training who attends or assists in childbirth in hospitals, birthing centers, and private homes
Psychiatrist	a physician who treats mental and emotional problems and illnesses
Psychologist	a person who completes a graduate program, clinical training, and an internship in human psychology and can provide psychotherapy and counseling
Social Worker	a person who is a certified social worker (CSW) or licensed clinical social worker (LCSW) has the education and training needed to help people work through their problems through counseling

1-5 You and your baby may need to see various types of health care providers.

Evaluating Health Care Providers

When evaluating a health care provider, you can find the answers to these questions to help you get to know the provider better.

❖ What is the provider's educational and training background?

❖ What experience has the person had in providing the type of service and treatment you need?

❖ Is the provider certified and licensed to provide services in your state?

❖ What are the person's areas of treatment or expertise?

❖ Do former and current patients speak well of the provider?

❖ Is the provider affiliated with a hospital, clinic, or group practice that is available to you and your family?

❖ Is the provider available to give care when you need it? Who covers in the provider's absence?

1-6 These questions can help you evaluate and choose qualified health care providers to meet your needs.

A Visit to the Public Aid Office

Many of the services you need may come from the public aid office. This office may have different names, depending on where you live. Some of these names are the Department of Health and Human Services, the Department of Social and Rehabilitative Services (SRS), and the Department of Child and Family Services (DCFS). Whatever its name, you can apply for federal aid at this office.

To start this process, call the public aid office. Ask where the office is located and request an appointment. Find out what documents you need to bring to your first appointment. See Figure 1-7

Checklist: Applying for Public Assistance

You will likely need to bring the following papers with you when you apply for assistance at the public aid office. Some of this same information may be required by other sources of assistance.

_____ Driver's license or photo identification card (state ID or school ID)

_____ Social Security card and Medicaid cards

_____ Birth certificates or baptismal certificates

_____ Physician's statements, verification of pregnancy, medical records

_____ School records, diploma, GED certificate

_____ Pay stubs and employment records

_____ Proof of income and money from jobs, loans, relatives, gifts

_____ Proof of scholarship, tuition, loans, and education expenses

_____ Marriage certificate, divorce decree, death certificates, military service records

_____ Child support orders

_____ Rent receipts and utility bills

_____ Title, registration, contract, and payment book on motor vehicles you own

_____ Records of bank or credit union accounts

_____ Policies for life or health insurance

_____ Paid or unpaid doctor, hospital, or dental bills

_____ Records of any property sales or purchases you've made within the past 3 years

1-7 Use this checklist to help you gather the documents and information you may need to take with you if you apply for assistance.

for a sample checklist. Be sure to keep your appointment. If you must cancel, be sure to do so in advance.

Once you arrive at the public aid office, you will start the process of applying for aid. It may take several appointments to complete this process. The process varies from state to state, but often has three basic steps. These include

1. a screening appointment with a human services officer. At your first visit, this person will ask some basic questions about you, your baby, and your baby's father. These questions may include where you live, your income, age, marital status, education, and job history. See Figure 1-8. The human services officer is building your file for the next person you will see. In some cases, this person may be able to arrange temporary help to meet an immediate need for food or medical care.

2. an appointment with an eligibility specialist. This person will look over your paperwork and interview you. He or she will tell you what, if any, aid you can receive. This may include the following types of assistance: cash, medical care, child care, housing, and food. The specialist can also explain what you must do to qualify for this help.

3. a meeting with your caseworker. If you qualify for aid, a caseworker will be assigned to your case. This person will be your primary contact for whatever aid you receive. He or she will counsel you and supervise your case as long as you receive assistance. During this time, you are expected to stay in close contact with the public aid office. You will meet with your caseworker from time to time. You must also let him or her know when your situation changes. See Figure 1-9 for a list of changes you should report. Your caseworker can also direct you to other help you might need. This might include help with your education, job training, housing, counseling, legal aid, and child care. This person should be well aware of services in the community. This makes him or her a good person to ask for referrals.

Questions You May Be Asked

When you apply for public aid, you will be asked many questions. You may not want to answer very personal questions, but you may be required to do so in order to receive the help you need. The following are examples of questions you may be asked.

✤ Who are you? You will need to give your full name, address, phone number, Social Security number, and date of birth. You may need your birth certificate. After the baby is born, you'll need to provide the baby's birth certificate and Social Security number, too.

✤ What is your medical history? Be ready to answer questions about your health and habits. Be honest about whether you smoke or use alcohol or drugs. You will be asked about medical conditions that affect you or your family. Describe illnesses, injuries, surgeries, and medicines you have had in the past. You may also be asked about the medical history of the father and his family.

✤ What is your financial situation? You will be asked how much money or income you have and where it comes from. List benefits you currently receive such as Medicaid, cash assistance, food stamps, or other support. Keep receipts, pay stubs, and bills as proof of your income and expenses. Describe any property, such as a vehicle, you own.

✤ What is your education and job status? You will be asked the name of your school. The public aid office may talk with someone at your school to verify you are enrolled. If you are working, you must also give the name of your employer. You may be required to stay in school, be employed, or enroll in a job training program to receive assistance.

✤ What services or assistance do you need? You will be asked to describe your situation and what help you think you need. Bring bills and receipts to use as proof of expenses and living costs.

✤ Who is the father of the baby and what help can he offer? In most cases, you will be required to identify the father and describe your relationship with him. He will be legally obligated to provide child support. If you receive public aid, this support may be used to repay the government for the help you're receiving. You will be asked his full name, birth date, Social Security number, address, and phone number. Give whatever information about the father you can. This will help you get the assistance you need.

1-8 If you apply for assistance, your caseworker may ask you many personal questions such as these.

Changes in Circumstance You Must Report

You will need to contact your caseworker at the public aid office to report certain changes in your life. These include the following:

❖ new address or phone number

❖ change in income

❖ marriage, separation, or divorce

❖ changes in employment status

❖ pregnancy

❖ development of serious health problems by you or your child

❖ changes in your household—people move in or out of your household or the relationship changes between you and others in your household

❖ change in your housing costs

❖ a death or disability occurs in your family

1-9 To remain eligible for aid, people on public assistance are required to contact their caseworkers about these life changes.

Using the Phone to Find What You Need

Using the telephone can save you time and footwork. See Figure 1-10. You can use the phone to gather information and set appointments. The following guidelines can help you make every telephone call count:

☛ Before making your call, write a list of questions you want to ask. Think about what questions you may be asked, and be prepared to answer them. Writing a list of these questions and answers may help.

☛ Have paper and pen handy. When you make an appointment, write a note to yourself. Include the name of the person you're to see, as well as the address, phone number, date, and time of the appointment. Add any other information you receive to this note. This will help you remember what you need to know.

☛ Ask for the name of each person you talk with. Make a note of the name, as well as the date and time of the call. In a follow-up call, you may need to ask for that person again or give his or her name. This can verify you have called before. It may also help a new person who takes your call locate information you have already given. This way you do not have to start from scratch each time you call.

☛ Speak clearly and slowly so you will be understood. Talk loudly enough to be heard. Avoid using slang the other person might not understand. Don't curse or use threatening language, even if you're upset.

☛ Be polite but firm in getting the answers you need. Keep trying until you find out what you want to know or reach the person you want to talk with. This is not always easy, but don't give up!

Keeping It Together

Your notes and important papers are only useful if you know where they are and can access them easily. If you haven't done so already, now is a good time to start a notebook or filing system.

Store your important papers in one place—a notebook, basket, or file box—where you can always find them. Start a folder for each main area. For instance, you might have a folder for each of the following: school papers, public aid, work, and medical papers. File each note and paper in the folder where it belongs. This allows you to locate information quickly. (You will learn more about keeping records safe and handy in Chapter 3.)

It's also a good idea to keep a master list of resources in your area. Update the list once in a while so it will always be current. Keeping track of what you know helps you make this information work for you.

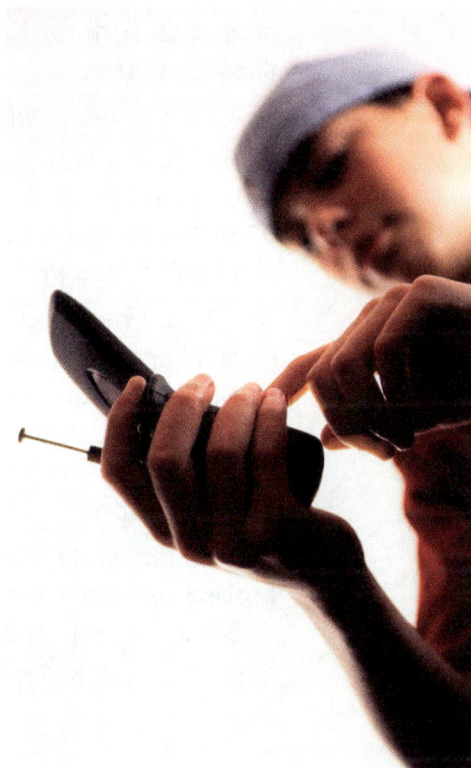

1-10 Compare the time and effort used to set an appointment by phone and the time and effort it takes to travel to the office and do it in person.

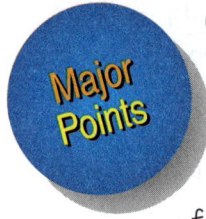

☞ Getting the help you need is one of your first tasks when facing an unplanned pregnancy. Your well-being and your baby's welfare depend on it. There are many places you can look for this help.

☞ Telephone hot lines may be a valuable resource for you. Many provide round-the-clock counseling, as well as referrals to other agencies you might contact for help. You can also turn to the Internet for information.

☞ Many government agencies offer programs that may be of help to you. The Department of Health and Human Services offers many public aid and public service programs. The GED program is available through the Department of Education. The Department of Housing may be able to help you find low-income or subsidized housing.

☞ Social service programs and religious organizations are other places to turn for help. Contact these agencies to learn what help they can offer.

☞ Clinics, hospitals, and medical groups are places to look for the health care you need. Take your time when choosing a health care facility and provider. Ask questions about the types of care provided at different facilities. You may want to find out the qualifications of the health care professionals who will treat you, too.

☞ If you visit the public aid office to apply for assistance, remember to take with you all the papers and information needed. It will likely take a few visits for you to complete the application process. This may consist of a meeting with a human services officer, a meeting with an eligibility specialist, and a meeting with your caseworker.

☞ You can use the phone to gather information you will need. Making appointments by phone is helpful, too. Remember to take notes when making important phone calls. File these notes and your important papers so you can find them easily when you need them.

Chapter 2
Understanding
Legal Matters

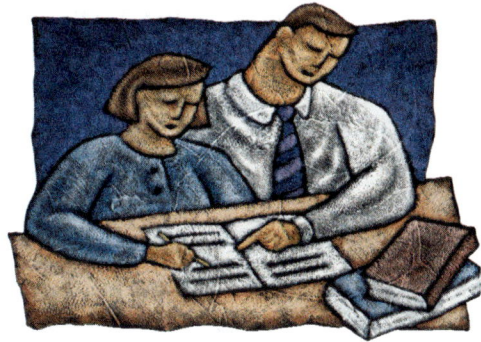

Teen pregnancy brings with it many decisions. No matter which option you choose regarding your pregnancy, there are legal matters to consider. If you become a parent, you will take on new legal status along with your new responsibilities. You may need to be aware of laws regarding family matters, such as marriage, parenting, and child support. If you choose not to parent, these options have legal aspects, too. Now is a good time to learn about your legal rights and responsibilities when it comes to these decisions.

You and Your Partner

When teens choose parenting, both partners must decide how this will change their relationship. Some couples choose to marry. Others decide to live together and share parenting responsibilities. Still other teen parents live apart. In many of these families, the mother takes the primary role and may be the only parent involved in the child's life. More often now than in the past, though, young fathers are choosing to play a major role even when they don't live with their children. No matter what their family situation, teen parents have legal issues to consider.

Living Together

In response to pregnancy, many teen couples choose to stay together. Some choose to live together rather than marry. It may seem easier and less complicated to do this. Often it is even more complicated, though. Under the law, couples who live together lack the legal status of married couples. This matters most when it comes to the following:

- ☛ property rights. Who owns what? Who gets what if the relationship ends? (Try to avoid owning any items together unless you are married. Settling property disputes can be difficult if the relationship ends.)
- ☛ housing. Whose home is it? Who gets it if the partnership ends?
- ☛ expenses. Who pays for what?
- ☛ child care, support, and custody. Who will be responsible for the well-being of the children during the relationship and if it ends?

Before moving in together, discuss these points with your partner. Be sure you agree on these important issues. A verbal agreement may not be enough, though. If you separate, one of you might decide not to carry out the terms you agreed upon before. For the strongest protection against this, you and your partner can create a written agreement. When prepared properly, a written agreement is legally binding. This means it can be upheld in court if needed. A lawyer can help you create this type of agreement.

Marriage

Some teen parents choose to marry. They become partners, both in an emotional and legal sense. Marriage gives more rights and protection under the law than living together does. See Figure 2-1. A married couple is seen as a unit for most legal and business matters. They can file a joint tax return and open a joint bank account. After they marry, both people jointly own any money and property they gain.

Spouses also have other legal rights. One spouse can often include the other in job-related health insurance and other benefits. In an emergency, a spouse can make decisions about his or her partner's medical care. After a death, the spouse will inherit at least part of the person's estate. Social Security will also pay benefits to a person's spouse after he or she has died.

You can learn more about deciding whether to marry in another title in this series, <u>Understanding Your Changing Life</u>. This is a serious decision. Take your time. If you choose to marry, find out what your state laws are, because marriage laws vary by state. Many states require that you

- ☞ be at least a certain age to marry (set by the state)
- ☞ have your parents' permission if you're under the legal age set by the state
- ☞ are married to only one person at a time
- ☞ cannot marry a blood relative
- ☞ must be able to freely consent to the marriage

To marry, you will need a marriage license. You and your partner can apply for this at the county clerk's office. Both of you must appear in person and pay a small fee. You must also provide proof of your identity. This might be a birth certificate, driver's license, or state ID card. Some states require a medical exam and blood tests. Others set a waiting period between getting the license and the time you can marry. Your county clerk's office will know what your state requires.

2-1 Married teens have more legal rights than those who just live together. Marriage also promotes a more secure relationship.

A marriage license is valid for a set time, often six months. During this time, it is legal for the two of you to wed. A member of the clergy, justice of the peace, judge, or clerk of the court can conduct the marriage ceremony. This official will sign the certificate and file it with the county clerk's office.

Contact the county clerk's office for a copy of the marriage certificate. It is wise to have at least one official copy for your records. You may need this certificate to change your name or marital status for business matters.

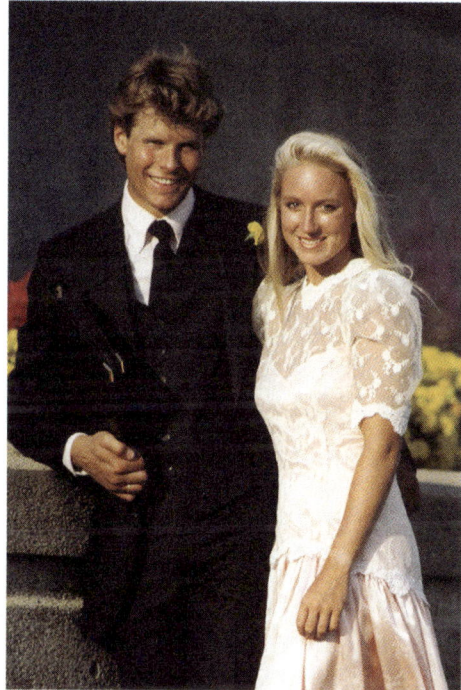

When a couple marries, the changing of last names may be an issue. In the past, husbands kept their last names and wives took their husband's last names. Most married couples still follow this pattern. However, there are other patterns, too. A wife (or both partners) may use both partners' last names joined by a hyphen. In some cases, a husband may take his wife's last name. A couple should decide about this before they marry.

If any name changes will occur, the names must be changed on important documents and records. A change of name and marital status are often required for the following:

- driver's license
- Social Security card
- voter registration
- passport
- bank accounts
- credit cards
- insurance policies
- work and school records
- medical records

When a married person keeps the same name, fewer changes are needed. The person may need to notify his or her employer, insurance company, bank, and creditors. This is especially true if the person is adding the spouse to a benefit plan, insurance policy, bank account, or credit account. People on public aid must also tell their caseworkers of a marriage.

Common Law Marriage

In some states, it is legal for two people to be married without a marriage license or a ceremony. This is known as a common law marriage. For this to happen, a couple must live together as husband and wife. Just living in the same house does not result in a common law marriage. Couples are seen as married only if they present themselves in public as husband and wife.

Common law marriage is not a new idea. It was started long ago. In many rural areas, one judge traveled among many counties, spending time in each. It might take months for the judge to return to the county where a couple lived. For this reason, couples were allowed to live as husband and wife. These marriages were recognized as legal. Times have changed, but this option is still legal in some areas. See Figure 2-2.

A common law marriage provides the same legal rights and protections as any other marriage. It also requires legal steps if the couple wishes to end the marriage.

Where Is Common Law Marriage Legal?

- District of Columbia
- Alabama
- Colorado
- Iowa
- Kansas

- Montana
- Oklahoma
- Rhode Island
- South Carolina
- Texas

2-2 Currently, the District of Columbia and nine states recognize common law marriage.

Living Separate Lives

Suppose you and your partner (or former partner) are going to be parents. This doesn't mean the two of you are ready to marry. It also doesn't mean you would make good spouses for each other. You may not be. In this case, the two of you may choose to live separate lives. If so, you will face many legal issues. These include parental responsibilities, paternity, and decisions about the roles each of you will play in your child's life. You will read more about these topics later in this chapter. (You can also learn more by reading another title in this series, Understanding Your Changing Life.)

Breaking the Marriage Contract

Since marriage is a legal contract, it can only be broken by legal means. If a couple wants to end their marriage, they have three options. These are annulment, legal separation, and divorce. These options differ in major ways. Each of them is costly and can be complicated. Ending a marriage is not easy emotionally, either. It can cause pain for both spouses and their children.

An annulment is a court decree that dissolves a marriage by declaring it null and void. It makes it as though the marriage never occurred. This is usually done fairly soon after the marriage begins. There are only a few reasons why an annulment can be granted. These vary from state to state. The court does rule on child support, custody, and visitation. It also helps divide the couple's property fairly.

In a legal separation, spouses make an agreement to live apart. This doesn't end their marriage. Instead, it sets rules for both people to follow while they lead their own lives. This protects both partners. Couples often separate as they decide whether to divorce. After separating, a couple may choose to resume their marriage. They might also decide to keep living apart without divorcing. This may work well for them as long as neither person wants to remarry.

In a legal separation, the couple must create a settlement. This must be approved by the court. The settlement outlines the rights and obligations of both people. It covers the following: child support, custody and visitation; financial support; bills and debts; and the division of property.

Laws about legal separation vary from state to state. A lawyer can tell you about the laws in your state. Ask him or her to explain how legal separation differs from a divorce. Your lawyer can advise you which option is best for you.

A divorce is the formal end of a marriage. A couple must file for divorce in the state where they live. In most cases, legal help is needed to file for divorce. The partners must create and agree to a permanent settlement. This will cover the division of property, money, bills, and debts. It should also state terms for custody, child support, and visitation. Once the divorce decree is approved by the court, the marriage is ended.

Some states require a couple to prove there are acceptable reasons, or grounds for divorce. See Figure 2-3. This type of divorce is a fault divorce. Other states allow no-fault divorce. This means a couple can end their marriage by mutual consent without having grounds or proving fault. If you're considering divorce, find out what the laws are in your state.

Before ending a marriage, it may help to seek counseling. This can let both partners explore whether they can work to save the marriage. If they still choose to end the marriage, counseling can prepare them for this. It can help them work through their feelings about it. Parents can also learn to guide and nurture their children through this process. A trusted adult may be able to help you find a good counselor. You could ask your health care provider or a religious leader, too.

If you want to end your marriage, you will need to seek legal help. This will help you get a fair settlement and protect your legal rights. (You can read more about finding legal help later in this chapter.)

Grounds for Breaking the Marriage Contract

In some states, a couple can't divorce unless they can prove they have grounds, or reasons. Acceptable reasons for a fault divorce vary from state to state. The most common include the following on the part of the partner:

- insanity
- life-term prison sentence
- threats of violence
- being married to two or more people at once
- inability to perform sexually
- fraud
- desertion
- cruelty
- adultery
- drunkenness
- drug addiction
- nonsupport
- mental or physical abuse
- irreconcilable differences

2-3 Grounds for breaking the marriage contract are similar in every state.

The Law and Your Child

Suppose you choose to parent. No matter what relationship you and your partner have, you will both become parents of the same child. Each of you has rights and responsibilities when it comes to your child. Parenthood can bring with it many legal issues. This is especially true for those who are not married. You will need to learn more about the legal matters involving your child. This will help you protect her legal rights, as well as your own.

Parental Rights and Responsibilities

As a parent, you may wonder what your rights and responsibilities are. Many of your rights are protected under the law. Some of these include the following:

- ☞ the right to raise your child by your own values and ideas
- ☞ the right to choose where you will live and raise your child
- ☞ the right to make important choices about his schooling, religious beliefs, moral training, health care, and lifestyle
- ☞ the right to guide and discipline your child
- ☞ the right to speak as your child's legal representative if he must go to court
- ☞ the right to choose a lawyer for him should one be needed

These rights are protected as long as your behavior is within the law. For instance, you can't punish your child in a way that is abusive. The courts can take away your rights if your child's life or well-being is in danger. This can also happen if you show you cannot make appropriate choices regarding your child's welfare.

With your rights come certain responsibilities. Your child needs you to protect and care for him. Legally, you must meet these responsibilities to keep your rights as a parent. You are responsible for the following:

- ☞ making every effort to meet your child's physical needs. These include food, shelter, clothing, and health care. You may need to seek assistance if you cannot afford these things.

- ☛ overseeing your child's education. You must make sure he attends school daily and has the supplies he needs.

- ☛ providing adequate supervision for your child at all times. It is illegal to leave your baby or child unattended or home alone. (In many states, this law applies to all children under age 12.) If you must be away from your child, you must arrange for someone to stay with him until you return.

- ☛ protecting your child from danger. You are expected to make his environment as safe as possible. You must take needed precautions to keep him safe at all times.

- ☛ providing financial and emotional support for your child until he reaches the age of adulthood. In most states, this age is 18 years.

The Importance of Fathers

Today more pregnant teens choose to raise their babies as single parents than in the past. More than 70 percent of teen mothers are not married when they give birth. These children are not assured a relationship with their fathers. This trend raises serious questions about a father's role in his child's life.

Fathers are important to their children. See Figure 2-4. This fact is well supported by years of research. When fathers are involved in their children's lives, the children are more likely to

- ☛ perform better in school
- ☛ have more healthy relationships with others
- ☛ develop more self-esteem
- ☛ stay away from gangs and crime

A father's financial support adds to his child's well-being, too. This support enables the mother to meet the child's basic needs. It can keep the child out of poverty and improve the quality of her life.

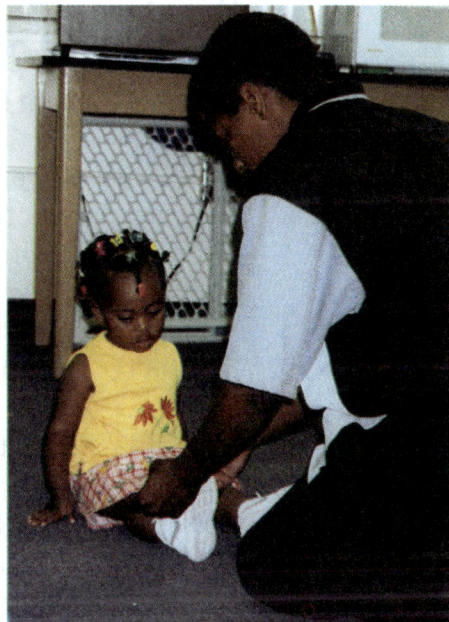

2-4 Fathers can provide physical care for their children as well as emotional and financial support.

It takes two parents to create a child. Both parents should take responsibility for raising her. Even if they don't live together, both parents can guide and support her. Children tend to do best in life when both parents are involved in their lives. When one parent is absent from their lives, children feel this loss. This is true even if they never knew this absent parent.

Unfortunately, though, some men choose not to be involved with their children. Even when ordered by the court to pay child support, some men do not comply. They may also decide not to connect emotionally with their children. If your child's father is not as involved as you would like, it can be frustrating. You can't force him to have a relationship with his child, however. This is his responsibility. You might try staying in contact with his family, though. This can encourage him to get involved. Even if he still doesn't want to be involved, your child will know her other family. This can be important to her.

As the mother, you play a role in influencing his decision. Your actions and attitudes can make it easier or harder for him to be a father. The person this affects most is your child. For her sake, encourage him to be a good father. Work with him to raise her. Ask for his input and support his positive efforts. Let him share the responsibility and rewards of parenting.

In a few cases, there are serious reasons to avoid the father of your baby. This is true if he has been abusive to you or others in the past. His involvement may make you fear for the life or safety of you or your child. If so, discuss this with a lawyer. The court may be able to help protect you. Even if the court still enforces visitation, this can be done in the safest way possible.

Unless this is the case, think carefully before you deny your child a relationship with her father. You may not be interested in seeing him, but he is the father of your child. Your child deserves a chance to get to know her father. She needs the opportunity to bond with him. If she develops a close relationship with him, this will be good for her.

Having the father involved will also help you. It means you're not left to do everything on your own. The more you can work with him and his family, the more help they can be. Allow the father to have as large a role as he is willing to play. This will help you lower the amount of stress and responsibility you carry alone.

A father who connects with his child also benefits. First, he has the joy of being a parent and forming a relationship with her. This can be satisfying and fulfilling for him. If he takes his role seriously, he may be more likely to keep a job and avoid criminal behavior. This will happen if he wants to support his child both financially and emotionally. Being a father can increase his self-esteem, too.

Establishing Paternity

Paternity means the biological fatherhood of a child. Suppose a couple is married and the woman gives birth. Legally, it is assumed the husband is the child's father. For couples who aren't married, though, fatherhood is not assumed. It must be admitted by the father or proven through testing.

Establishing paternity is important. Your child deserves to have a legal father and know who his father is. He is also legally entitled to certain benefits through his father. These include present and future benefits from the following:

- ☛ child support payments
- ☛ health insurance coverage
- ☛ military dependents' benefits (if his father is in the armed forces)
- ☛ dependent's benefits from workers' compensation, pension programs, and life insurance policies
- ☛ inheritance rights
- ☛ Social Security benefits (if his father dies or becomes disabled)

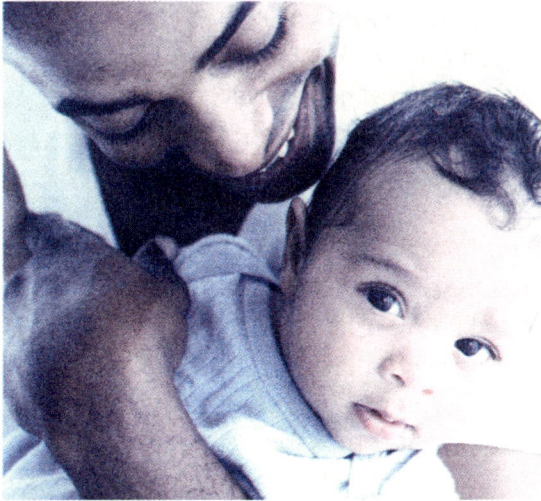

This newborn will benefit greatly by having his father involved from birth.

2-5

The best and easiest way to establish paternity is for the father to admit the child is his. Next, he would file the proper papers with the court. This can be done at the birth facility when the baby is born. To do this, both parents sign the forms the birth facility provides. It's good to do this at birth. A father is more likely to be involved with his child if he is in the child's life from the start. See Figure 2-5.

Most often when parents are not wed, the father's name cannot appear on the baby's birth certificate until his paternity is declared. He can do this at or after the birth. The papers he would need to file are available through the birth facility or the court. When paternity is declared, his name may be added to the birth certificate. If you have questions about this, ask your lawyer.

In some cases, a man might not think he is the child's father. This is often true if he and the baby's mother were only together a short time or each saw other people. It might not be known which man is the father. In other cases, a man might not want to be a father. This might also lead him to deny paternity.

If a man denies he is the father, the mother can file a paternity suit in court. She can hire a lawyer to file this case. This option is costly, though. Instead, she could work with her local Child Support Enforcement (CSE) office. This government office can help her find the father (if needed) and establish paternity. Then the CSE office can help her file a child support case with the court. It can also enforce the collection of child support owed by the father.

To establish paternity, the CSE office can ask the court to order a paternity test. The test involves taking cells from both the man and the baby. This can be done by a blood test or a tissue test (often a swab from the inside of the mouth). The genetic makeup of the man's cells and the baby's cells are then compared. This can reveal whether the man is the child's father. These tests are very accurate. They can exclude a man who is not the father. These tests can also determine the likelihood that a man is the father. A paternity test is accepted by the court as legal proof of paternity.

If you receive public aid, the law says you must cooperate in this process. You must help find the father and establish paternity. You must give your caseworker and the CSE office all the information you have to help them do this. If you fear for the safety or well-being of you and your child, tell your caseworker. In such a case, you may not be required to give this information. The court can choose not to pursue child support if this might endanger mother or child.

Even if you don't receive public aid, the CSE office can help you with locating the father and establishing paternity, as well as seeking and enforcing a child support order. Check with your state's office to find out what, if any, fees you must pay.

It's best to establish paternity legally as early as possible, even if you and the baby's father are still together. This protects your child's rights in case you and your baby's father break up at some time in the future.

In most cases your child would benefit from having paternity established. It can be a long process, but it is worth it. Settling paternity issues also gives the father legal rights and responsibilities as a parent. These may encourage him to play a positive role in his child's life.

Custody and Visitation

Child custody refers to the rights that parents who live apart are given by the court regarding their child. Two types of custody are legal and physical. Legal custody means having the right to make major decisions about your child's welfare. These include choices about school, religion, and health care. Physical custody is the right to have your child live with you and to provide physical care for her. A parent with this type of custody is called the residential parent. One who does not have physical custody or live with the child is called a nonresidential parent. You may see the terms <u>custodial parent</u> and <u>noncustodial parent</u> used instead. These terms have the same meaning. See Figure 2-6.

If only one parent has legal and physical custody, this is called sole custody. A second custody arrangement is called joint custody. This means sharing one or both types of custody with the child's other parent. In joint custody, the court grants each parent certain rights. It may also set the amount of time the child spends with each parent.

Custody can be a complex matter. This often depends on how much conflict there is between the parents. If they get along well, it may be easy to make the custody decisions together and have them approved by the court. If not, each parent may have to present his or her case and let the court decide. The court's primary concern in custody cases is the best interest of the child. This should be the parents' concern as well.

Child Custody Terms

- ❖ **Child custody**—the rights that parents who live apart are given by the court regarding their child.
- ❖ **Custodial parent**—parent who has physical custody and lives with his or her child.
- ❖ **Joint custody**—custody arrangement in which both parents share one or both types of custody (physical and legal).
- ❖ **Legal custody**—type of custody that allows a parent to make decisions regarding a child's welfare.
- ❖ **Noncustodial paren**t—parent who does not have physical custody or live with his or her child.
- ❖ **Nonresidential parent**—parent who does not have physical custody or live with his or her child.
- ❖ **Physical custody**—type of custody that gives a parent the right to have the child live with him or her and the responsibility to provide the child's physical care.
- ❖ **Residential parent**—parent who has physical custody and lives with his or her child.
- ❖ **Sole custody**—custody arrangement in which only one parent has physical and legal custody of a child.

2-6 Child custody can be a complex issue. You would need legal help to create a custody agreement.

Visitation rights are the court-approved rights of a parent to see his or her child. Some parents may be able to work out a visitation plan together. If so, the plan will need to be approved by the court. Otherwise, the terms of visitation can be set by the court. The court must also approve any changes to the terms.

If the parents can't agree, this can make things more difficult. To avoid problems, they should be sure specific terms of visitation are set. The court order should state the exact days and times for visitation. It should avoid terms that are not specific, such as <u>reasonable visitation</u>. This kind of wording doesn't protect the rights of either parent.

Once a visitation plan is in effect, both parents must follow it exactly. Neither parent can deny the other the visitation ordered by the court. This is true whether child support has or has not been paid. Parents can be held in contempt of court for not allowing visitation to take place. Neither parent can fail to return a child when the visit is scheduled to end. Parents can be charged with kidnapping if they fail to return a child as required by the visitation order. If parents want to change the visitation plan, they must appeal to the court.

Child Support

Both parents are financially responsible for supporting their child. Married parents are a unit. If they both work, they share the costs of raising the child. Matters are more complex when parents live apart, though. The residential parent should not be the only one to pay the costs of raising a child. The law states the nonresidential parent must support the child, too.

A nonresidential parent may be ordered by the court to make child support payments. These are payments to the residential parent for the support of a child. This money must be used to pay for food, clothing, health care, child care, education, and other items the child needs. Child support is not to be used for a parent's personal expenses.

In a few cases, both parents agree on the amount of child support to be paid. The nonresidential parent may start paying this amount voluntarily. This is the ideal way to arrange child support. It is still best to have the plan approved and ordered by the court. This makes it legally binding.

In most cases, though, the court sets the amount of child support to be paid. The court bases its ruling on guidelines set by the state government. The court will take into account both parents' incomes and the number of children they have. Once the court rules, the nonresidential parent must start paying as ordered.

Even with a court order, collecting child support can be difficult. Payments are often random and unreliable. Many parents do not pay the full amount ordered. Some do not pay at all.

If this occurs, you may want to contact the local CSE office. The CSE staff can help you collect child support you have been awarded by the court. This may be done through a wage withholding order or garnishment. These are court orders sent to the nonresidential parent's employer. They require the employer to deduct child support payment from each paycheck the parent earns. This amount is then sent to the court to be given to the residential parent for the support of the child.

If you can't find the other parent, the CSE staff can help locate him or her. This is easier to do now than it once was. Recent reform of the public aid system has made it easier to collect child support that has been ordered by the court. See Figure 2-7.

Collecting child support may seem like a hassle, but it is your child's right. This money can give your child what he needs. More than that, it proves his father is taking at least a small amount of responsibility for his care. This may matter a great deal to your child when he's older.

Adoption and the Law

When faced with pregnancy, not all teens decide to parent. Some choose the legal process of adoption. This allows them to transfer their role as parents to other adults, called the adoptive parents. The adoptive parents then become the child's legal parents. They care for her and raise her as their own. The parents to whom a child was born are called birthparents. They can feel secure their child will be well cared for in her new home.

Changes in Public Aid Related to Child Support

❖ **The National New Hire Reporting System** establishes a Federal Case registry and National Directory of New Hires to track parents who are not paying child support across state lines. This makes it easier to find absent parents. The law also simplifies direct witholding of child support payments from wages.

❖ **The Streamlined System for Establishing Paternity** makes it easier to establish paternity at the birth facility at the time of birth.

❖ **The Uniform Interstate Child Support Law** simplifies the collection of child support payments from absent parents who live in different states from their children.

❖ **The Tougher Penalties for Nonpayment** expands wage garnishment provisions. States may also seize the assets and property of nonpaying parents or require them to work. In addition, states may revoke the licenses (drivers, professional, recreational, and occupational) of parents who are behind with child support payments. Nonresidential parents of children on public aid may be required to enroll in job training programs if they are unemployed or can't afford to pay child support.

❖ **The Computerized Statewide Collections** provision requires states to establish central registries of child support orders, centralized collection and disbursement units, and speedier procedures for enforcing child support.

2-7 The public aid system has changed in ways that make it easier to collect child support payments from nonresidential parents.

Adoption can be a good option for pregnant teens who

- ☛ feel they are not ready to handle the ongoing responsibilities of parenthood
- ☛ believe a child needs to grow up in a home with two parents who are mature and ready for parenthood
- ☛ feel unable to properly care for a child for any reason

When considering adoption, you should know you have several choices. See Figure 2-8 for a brief summary. If you want to learn more about an agency adoption, contact an adoption agency near you. Ask your health care provider to refer you to one. This agency can tell you what you need to know. Visiting an agency doesn't mean you must

Adoption Options

Do you prefer an agency or independent adoption?

❖ An **agency adoption** is arranged by a state-licensed adoption agency. This agency would provide counseling, match you with an adoptive family, handle the legal steps, help you seek medical care, and support you through this process. Agencies also screen adoptive parents thoroughly to be sure they are fit to be parents.

❖ An **independent adoption** is a direct agreement between birthparents and adoptive parents. A doctor, lawyer, or other person might match the birthparents and adoptive parents. Both sets of parents should have lawyers to help them take care of the legal matters. An independent adoption may not include counseling and support services. There is also much less screening of adoptive parents in this type of adoption.

Do you want an open or closed adoption?

❖ An **open adoption** permits some degree of contact between birthparents and the adoptive family. Both sets of parents may meet and keep some type of ongoing contact. The birthparents and the adoptive parents decide together how much and what kinds of contact will occur between them. They will usually come to an agreement about this before the adoption.

❖ In a **closed adoption**, the birthparents and adoptive parents prefer to have no contact with each other. In this type of adoption, birthparents may or may not choose the adoptive family. Neither set of parents receives identifying information about the other. This protects the privacy of all concerned.

2-8   Adoption involves many important choices.

choose adoption. It just means you are seeking information. (See another title in this series, Understanding Your Changing Life, to learn more about the types of adoption and the adoption decision.)

In addition to these choices, some birthparents may also think about informal adoption. This means their child would live with someone else but not go through all the legal steps of adoption. Often, this person would be a relative. An informal adoption would not be recognized by the law. It won't give your child the same legal protection as other parenting options. See Figure 2-9 for more information on informal adoption.

Adoption is legal in every state, but the laws in each state may vary. Almost all states have laws that govern the following parts of the adoption process:

☞ pre-placement evaluation and home study of the adoptive parents

☞ waiting periods

☛ birthparent counseling

☛ consent of both birthparents

☛ opening of sealed adoption records when child reaches adulthood

A good adoption agency can explain the laws in your state. You can also contact the National Adoption Information Clearinghouse to learn more. This national agency offers adoption information to the public. Knowing the laws will help you understand the process and the options you have.

Birthparents' Legal Rights

As a birthparent, you have rights under the law. When you know your rights, you can make sure they are protected. This will also help you handle matters in the right way. Two of your main rights are described in the paragraphs that follow.

Informal Adoption

Suppose you have a family member whom you would like to take care of your child. For instance, it might be one of your parents, grandparents, aunts, cousins, or sisters. The child might live with this relative until you are ready to take care of him. This is called an *informal adoption*. Legally, no parenting rights have been transferred.

This arrangement will not give your child much legal protection. The person who is caring for him wouldn't have the same parenting rights you do. For example, your family member might not be able to provide health insurance for the child on his or her policy because the child is still legally your responsibility.

In this situation, you have two options to give your child more legal protection and rights.

❖ First, the primary caregiver may decide to formally adopt the child. This would mean you would transfer your parenting rights and responsibilities to the other person. He or she would become the child's legal parent. This is a permanent option.

❖ Second, the caregiver could become a temporary guardian under the law. This would not be a permanent choice, but it would allow you to resume parenting at a later time. It would also protect your child in the meantime.

If you are in an informal adoption arrangement, ask for legal advice about how to proceed. This will help you protect the legal rights and interests of each person involved.

2-9   Informal adoption is not recognized by the law and does not give the child the same kind of rights as adoption does.

➤ You have the right to make your own decision about adoption. As the birthparent, you can choose to plan an adoption for your child. This right might not apply if you are a registered member of a Native American tribe. In this case, the tribe might have to give its consent to the adoption. Otherwise, the choice belongs to you and the birthfather. Both of you are entitled to participate in all phases of the adoption plan.

Both birthparents must consent to an adoption before it can take place. In some states, the birthfather can sign consent papers at any time before the baby is born. His consent will become valid after the baby is born. The birthmother cannot give her consent until after the baby is born. This protects each person's right to change his or her mind before the adoption is finalized.

You must take legal steps to locate the birthfather and tell him of your plans. A lawyer can advise you about these steps and guide you through them. Suppose you can't find the birthfather or he doesn't respond. A hearing can be held to terminate his parenting rights. If he doesn't object to this or attend this hearing, his legal rights will be ended. Then you can go ahead with planning the adoption.

What if the birthfather doesn't consent to the adoption or he defends his parenting rights? In this case, an adoption may not be possible. Your lawyer can guide you through this process and inform you of your options in this situation. See Figure 2-10.

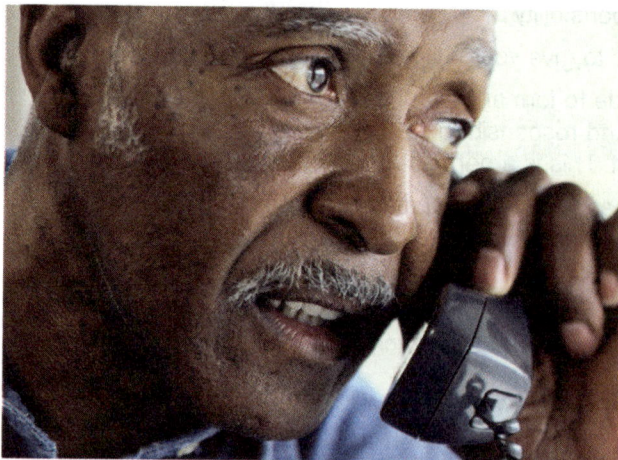

2-10 If you have legal questions regarding an adoption plan, your lawyer or legal aid representative should be able to advise you.

➤ You may have the right to have some of your expenses reimbursed. Financial concerns may be one of the reasons you might consider adoption. For instance, you may not be able to afford quality medical care. This care during pregnancy is vital. It protects the baby's health. The costs of delivery may also be beyond your means. In the adoption process, you might be charged fees for legal help or counseling.

The law may allow the adoptive parents or adoption agency to repay you for some of your expenses. These expenses must result from the pregnancy, delivery, and adoption. Each state decides which expenses can be repaid to the birthparents.

Most medical and delivery costs can be repaid. Some legal and counseling fees might be paid, too. In some states, there are other costs that can be reimbursed. Ask your lawyer what the law says would happen if you took this money and then changed your mind.

Keep in mind it's illegal for you to take any money not allowed by your state. This would be considered selling your baby, which is never legal. In many states, the court will order records of all expenses paid to anyone involved in the adoption. This includes birthparents, adoption agencies, lawyers, and others. These records ensure any amounts paid in an adoption are legal.

The Adoption Process

The adoption process includes all the legal steps you follow in an adoption. The process may vary depending on which type of adoption you choose. State laws may also affect this process. The basic legal steps are much the same for each adoption, though.

After the birth, both birthparents must sign a release form. (If the father's rights have been terminated, he would not need to sign any forms.) This form lets the adoptive parents or adoption agency take the baby from the birth facility. The release form doesn't make the adoption final. The birthparents can still change their minds. It just means they give their permission for someone else to take the baby from the birth facility.

The consent form is signed by both birthparents. This is the legal document that makes the adoption final. It gives the adoptive parents the rights to parent the child. This is often signed a few days after the baby is placed in the adoptive home. Waiting gives birthparents time to be sure of their choice. In some states, the birthparents can change their minds for 30 to 60 days from the time the consent form is signed. In other states, once the consent form is signed, the birthparents do not have the right to change their minds. If you're planning an adoption, you'll want to know what the laws are in your state.

The final adoption hearing is the last step. This is the court hearing at which the adoption is made complete. State law sets the amount of time between the signing of the consent form and this hearing. In most states, it is six months. At this court hearing, a final decree of adoption is granted by the court. This document states the adoption is final and legal.

Now the baby's original birth certificate will be placed under a court seal. A new one will be issued. It will name the adoptive parents as the baby's parents and contain the baby's new name. Under the law, the adoptive parents are now the child's parents. They have the same legal rights and duties as other parents.

Abortion and the Law

Some pregnant teens choose abortion. Abortion is the removal of an embryo or fetus from the uterus to end a pregnancy. This option involves many legal issues. The laws differ in each state. Most states restrict the length of time abortion is an option. In some states, abortion is not legal after the first three months of pregnancy. Others allow later abortions in some cases.

Some states require that certain information be given to women who want abortions. This may mean clinics must describe the procedure in detail. Often, they must also counsel women before and after abortions. Some states set a waiting period after a woman applies for abortion. This may last 24 or 48 hours. A woman can use this time to be sure about her choice.

Some states require a teen to tell her parents before she has an abortion. Others also require the parents' consent before a teen can have an abortion. These laws keep teens from having secret abortions. If a teen chooses an abortion, it can help her emotionally to have her parents' support.

If you're thinking about an abortion, find out about your state's laws. Be sure to check for the most recent legal developments in your state and at the federal level.

Abortion is a serious and final choice. Seek counseling before you decide. Discuss the matter with your partner, parents, and others you can trust. You may also want to consult your religious leader. An abortion can have both physical and emotional outcomes. As with all medical procedures, there are risks.

For some women, ending a pregnancy brings a heavy emotional burden. This is especially true when a teen feels the choice was not her own. Sometimes the partner or parents will push or force a teen to have an abortion. This can be devastating emotionally for her. Counseling after an abortion can help a woman resolve any negative feelings she has about what has happened.

Abortion should not be used as a form of birth control. There are many reliable ways to prevent pregnancy. (See another title in this series, Understanding Your Changing Life, to learn more about the abortion decision and birth control.)

Today many young people choose abstinence. This means postponing sex for now. They know this is the only sure way to prevent pregnancy. It also keeps them safe from sexually transmitted infections. Waiting can also help them focus on other aspects of their relationship. See Figure 2-11.

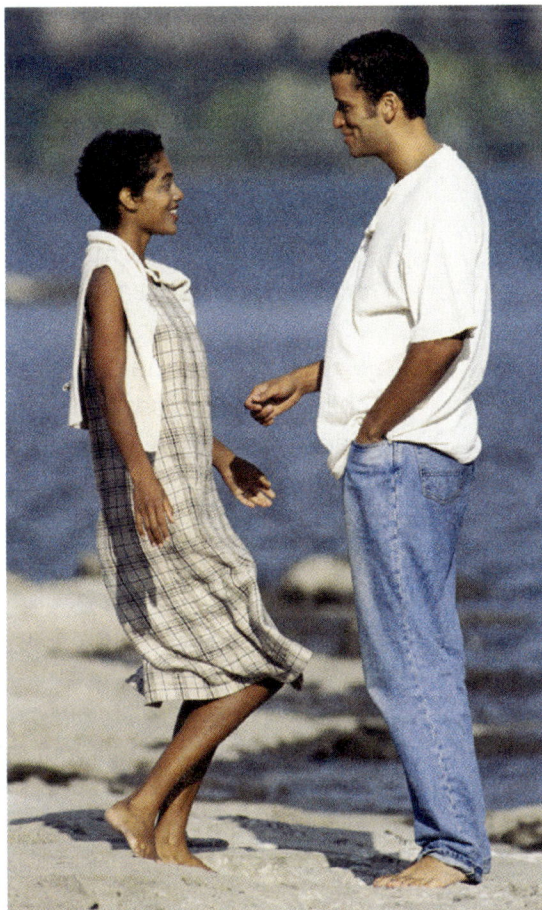

2-11 Abstinence can help you enjoy other aspects of your relationship. It can also prevent pregnancy and keep you safe from STIs.

Other Legal Issues

If you choose to parent, still other laws may affect your family. Laws against child abuse and domestic violence are meant to protect family members from harm. Laws about grandparents' rights, wills, and emancipation may matter to you, too. It's good to be aware of the laws in your state that relate to families. If you have questions about these issues, ask a lawyer for advice.

Child Abuse and Neglect

As a parent, you are required by law to care for and protect your child. This means protecting him from child abuse and neglect. You must make sure you never abuse or neglect your child. You must also keep a close watch to be sure no one else abuses or neglects him. This might include the other parent, child care providers, relatives, and friends who care for your child.

Child abuse is the intentional injury or pattern of injuries to a child. Three types of child abuse are physical, emotional, and sexual. Each of these is illegal. Child abuse is a crime that carries stiff legal penalties. It can even result in a prison term.

Child neglect means failing to meet a child's basic needs. Not giving a child the food, clothing, or loving attention he needs is neglect. Neglect is also illegal. It, too, has serious consequences.

State laws differ in exactly how they define child abuse and neglect. You can call your state's child abuse hot line to learn more. The hot line worker should have a copy of your state's legal definitions of child abuse and neglect. He or she should be able to explain what these laws mean.

You should also call the child abuse hot line if you believe your child has been abused or neglected. Report the incident and give all the facts you have. Be truthful even if the person is close to you. You must protect your child above all else.

In most states, the government will step in on behalf of children whose parents have abused or neglected them. In serious cases, the court can take a child away from his parents. The child might then go into the care of a relative or foster parents. In some cases, the court can even choose to terminate the parental rights of abusive parents. See Figure 2-12.

Stress or strong negative feelings may lead a parent to abuse or neglect a child. If you ever feel this might happen, seek help at once. Ask someone else to watch your child for you and take some time to yourself. What if there is no one else who can watch your child? Make sure he will be safe and then go into the other room for a few minutes. This will allow you to calm down and control your emotions. (To learn more about child abuse and neglect, see another title in this series, Understanding Your Changing Life.)

Domestic Violence

When Does the Court Terminate Parental Rights?

The court might decide to end your parental rights and take your child from you if you do any of the following:

* leave your child at home (or somewhere else) alone or leave your child with someone else and do not return within a reasonable amount of time
* fail to provide for your child's physical or emotional needs
* fail to enroll your child in school
* behave in a way that endangers your child's physical or emotional well-being or place your child in serious physical or emotional danger
* cause the injury or death of a child

2-12 These are common reasons the court terminates parental rights.

Domestic violence refers to harm a person does to someone close to him or her. This abuse can be physical, emotional, or sexual. It most often involves dating partners or spouses. This abuse can also occur between parent and child (child abuse) or two other relatives. No matter who is involved, domestic violence is a crime. It is illegal.

No one has the right to abuse you. If you are being abused, you have legal rights. State laws can protect you from domestic violence. Today, there are tougher laws against it. The penalties are more severe than in the past. More states now require the police to arrest the abuser after an incident of abuse.

In many states, you can file for an order of protection. This is a court order that sets specific terms to protect you from abuse. You can get one if your abuser lives with you now or did in the past. The name of the order may differ in your state, but its purpose will be the same.

This order may demand the person to have no contact with you and stay away from your home and job. It might grant you the possession of a shared home. The order might give you temporary custody of your child and demand that child support be paid.

Visit the office of your State's Attorney, located in your local courthouse. This person can tell you more about an order of protection and advise you what to do. You can also call a domestic violence hot line to learn more. Find out when and where you would go to seek this order. Once an order of protection is granted, an abuser must obey it. If the abuser breaks any of the terms of the order, he or she can be arrested. Call the police at once and show them the order. Keep a copy on you at all times.

Anti-stalking laws can also protect you. These laws make it a crime for someone to follow you around. Also, a person cannot make repeated, unwanted calls to your home or contact you in other ways you do not want. Again, call the State's Attorney or a domestic violence hot line to learn more about these laws. Call the police if someone violates an anti-stalking order. The stalker can be arrested for this.

If you want to leave an abusive partner, you can call a domestic violence hot line for help. This hot line can help you form a plan to leave or refer you to an emergency shelter where you and your children can be safe. (To learn more about domestic violence, see another title in this series, Understanding Your Changing Life.)

Grandparents' Rights

Almost all states grant grandparents the legal rights to see their grandchildren and participate in their lives. Laws vary greatly from state to state. Many teen parents want the grandparents to be close to their grandchildren. They encourage this special bond. See Figure 2-13.

In some cases, the grand-parents' relationship with the children is at risk. This may be true if the parents are unmar-ried, divorced, or remarried. It can also happen if the parents don't get along with the grandparents. For the most part, parents can limit visits to their children by others. Parents who keep the grand-parents away may feel they have good reason to do so.

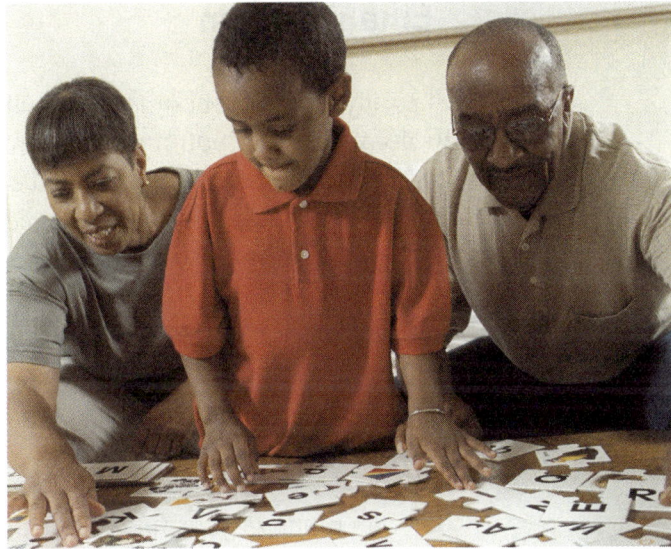

2-13 Most grandparents love their grandchildren and want to be involved in their lives.

At the same time, grandparents have rights. In serious cases, the court may step in to settle disputes over visitation and other rights of grandparents. This is done on a case-by-case basis. The court's concern is the best interest of the child. If this type of dispute arises in your family, seek legal counsel.

Wills

A will is a legal document that states how you want your matters settled after your death. In a sense, a will allows you to speak after you die. Your will can name an executor, a person who will carry out the terms of the will. You name the person whom you want to care for your children. This person is called a guardian. You can state how you want your property to be handled. It is wise to seek legal advice when writing a will.

This is especially true if your affairs tend to be complicated. If you die intestate (without a will), your property will be distributed according to state laws. The state will name a guardian for your children. This is why a will is important. It lets you make all the important decisions about your affairs and your children before your death.

Emancipation

Legally, you will become an adult at age 18. You would also be seen as an adult if you marry or enter active duty in the armed forces. In some cases, you might be able to petition the court to gain legal adult status. This is called emancipation. The laws about this vary from state to state.

Emancipation is granted through the court. You would need to sign papers asking the court to consider this option. Seek legal advice about whether this is a good option for you. The courts usually grant emancipation only if you

- ☞ can manage your finances from your own legal source of income
- ☞ show you can live on your own
- ☞ prove emancipation would be in your best interest

In most ways, an emancipated teen has the legal status of an adult. This person can enter binding contracts, sue or be sued, establish a home, and consent to medical care. The teen's parents no longer have the right to tell him or her what to do. The parents are also no longer required to provide financial support for the teen. An emancipated teen still does not have full adult rights, though. He or she cannot vote or buy tobacco and alcohol.

Emancipated teens may have problems if they apply for the Temporary Assistance to Needy Families (TANF). To receive aid, most teens are required to live with their parents. Some teens can prove they meet requirements to be exempt from this rule. These exemptions are granted on a case-by-case basis.

Obtaining Legal Services

You are most likely facing some of the legal issues described in this chapter. If so, you may need to seek legal help. You may wonder where to start. Finding good representation can take some effort.

Suppose you have been charged with a crime and can't afford a lawyer. In this case, the court will appoint a public defender to represent you. In all other legal matters, you will need to find your own legal help.

Cost is the main drawback to working with a private attorney. Most lawyers charge by the hour, and their rate is high. This cost may include the time you spend in the office, as well as time for their research, paperwork, phone calls, and other tasks. Fees can add up quickly, especially if your case is complex.

You may qualify for legal help through the legal aid association or legal aid society in your area. This agency may be able to offer you free or low-cost legal services. Whether you qualify is often based on your income and on the problem with which you need help. You can find the number for this office in the phone book under <u>Legal Aid</u> or <u>Legal Assistance Foundation</u>.

Whichever route you take, you may wonder how to choose a person to represent you. Figure 2-14 gives basic guidelines for obtaining legal help. It suggests when to seek legal help, how to find it, and what questions to ask. This figure also gives tips for making the most of legal services. You can use these guidelines as you choose legal help. Trust your instincts, too. You want someone with whom you will be comfortable.

If you don't qualify for help through the legal aid society, ask if the society can refer you to a legal aid hot line. In some areas, these hot lines serve low-income consumers. They can answer certain legal questions or refer you to low-cost legal services. You may also want to check out legal questions on the Internet. You can find answers to many questions online. A number of Web sites provide information about the law and legal issues. If you use a hot line or Web site, you may need to check with a lawyer or the legal aid society before following any advice you receive.

Obtaining Legal Help

How to Decide If You Need Legal Help

* Are you being sued or do you wish to sue someone?
* Are you party to a dispute involving large amounts of money or valuable property?
* Have you, your spouse, or your child been arrested or charged with a crime?
* Do you have problems with family legal issues such as separation, divorce, child support, custody, visitation, or property settlements?
* Do you feel your rights have been seriously violated on the job or in the marketplace?
* Are you entering a contract involving substantial money, assets, property, or labor?
* Do you want to make a will?
* Do you want to start a business?
* Do you need to declare bankruptcy?
* Have you been in a serious accident?

What to Ask When Choosing a Lawyer

* What type of law do you practice?
* How long have you been in practice?
* Where did you go to law school?
* Do you have other clients who would recommend you?
* Do you think I need legal representation and are you willing to take my case?
* Have you handled a case like mine before? What was the outcome?
* What cost can I expect for services I need? What types of payment arrangements can I make?

Where to Find Legal Advice

* Ask family and friends.
* Ask your caseworker, health care provider, or a hot line worker.
* Ask people at school, work, the community center, or any other organizations.
* Call the nearest legal aid society.
* Check the local bar association for referrals. (The bar association is a professional membership organization for lawyers. Most bar associations will offer referrals to the public.)

How to Make the Most of Legal Services

* Collect important facts and documents related to your case. These may include names, dates, addresses, dollar amounts, bills, receipts, and summaries of phone conversations. Bring this material to your first visit. Keep copies for yourself.
* Plan your questions in advance and take notes of your lawyer's advice.
* Keep informed on the progress of your case. Ask questions about anything you do not understand.
* Avoid unnecessary calls and appointments. Most lawyers charge by the hour.
* Tell your lawyer the whole truth. What you tell your lawyer is confidential. He or she needs to know all the facts to serve your interests.

2-14   You can use these guidelines to help you obtain and make the most of legal help.

Major Points

☛ Understanding legal matters means knowing your rights and responsibilities under the law. If you're not aware of your rights in a given situation, seek legal advice.

☛ You will need to learn about the legal aspects of your relationship with your partner. This is true whether you live together, are married, or live separate lives. Different laws apply to each of these arrangements.

☛ You may need to know about the laws that apply to breaking the marriage contract. Seek legal advice to learn more about annulment, legal separation, or divorce. You want to be sure your legal rights, and those of your children, are protected if you end your marriage.

☛ The law protects the children of parents who aren't married. These laws cover issues such as paternity, custody, visitation, and child support. Enforcing these laws can promote the important relationship between fathers and their children.

☛ Options such as adoption and abortion are also subject to the law. The laws regarding these issues vary from state to state. If you're interested in these options, you'll need to learn more about your state's laws.

☛ Several other issues that affect families are covered by law. These include child abuse and neglect, domestic violence, grandparents' rights, wills, and the emancipation of minors.

☛ You'll need to know where to find reliable legal services when you need them. A lawyer or legal aid society may be a good place to start when you need legal advice.

Chapter 3
Managing Money and Resources

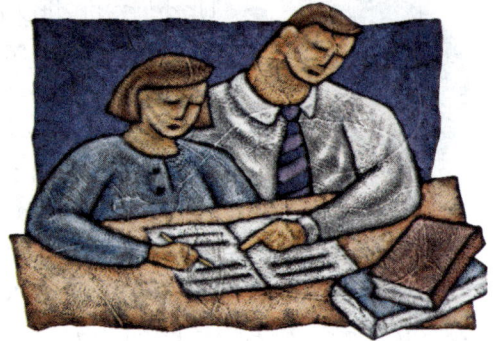

If you're like most teens, finances can be a problem. Chances are you have little or no money of your own. You may also have little practice in managing money. When pregnancy occurs, you may find you have even more expenses and bills. For these reasons, you need to learn how to manage your money and resources. These same skills will let you make the most of the help you get from your parents, partner, government, or other agencies.

Management means making wise use of what you have to meet your needs and wants. You can use management to help you reach your goals. A goal is a statement of what you want to accomplish. Setting goals allows you to achieve what's most important to you in life.

Identifying Your Resources

Resources are any and all tools you can use to reach your goals. For many, money is the first resource to come to mind. There are many others, though. Managing your resources wisely can help you reach more of your goals. There are three main types of resources. These are human, material, and community resources.

Human Resources

Human resources are those that come from within a person. You have many human resources. Some of these are your skills and talents. Your energy, experience, and knowledge are resources, too. Personal traits such as creativity can help you reach your goals. For more examples, see Figure 3-1. Which of the human resources listed are your strongest assets? Do you have others that are not on the list? Are there some you could develop?

At times, you can consider other people as your human resources. Friends and family members may offer their help, support, wisdom, skills, or time. Make the best use of these valuable resources. Accept offers from others to help you reach your goals.

Determination and Flexibility

Determination and flexibility are two key human resources. You can use them to help manage your other resources. You may have been born with these resources, or you may be able to develop them.

Human Resources

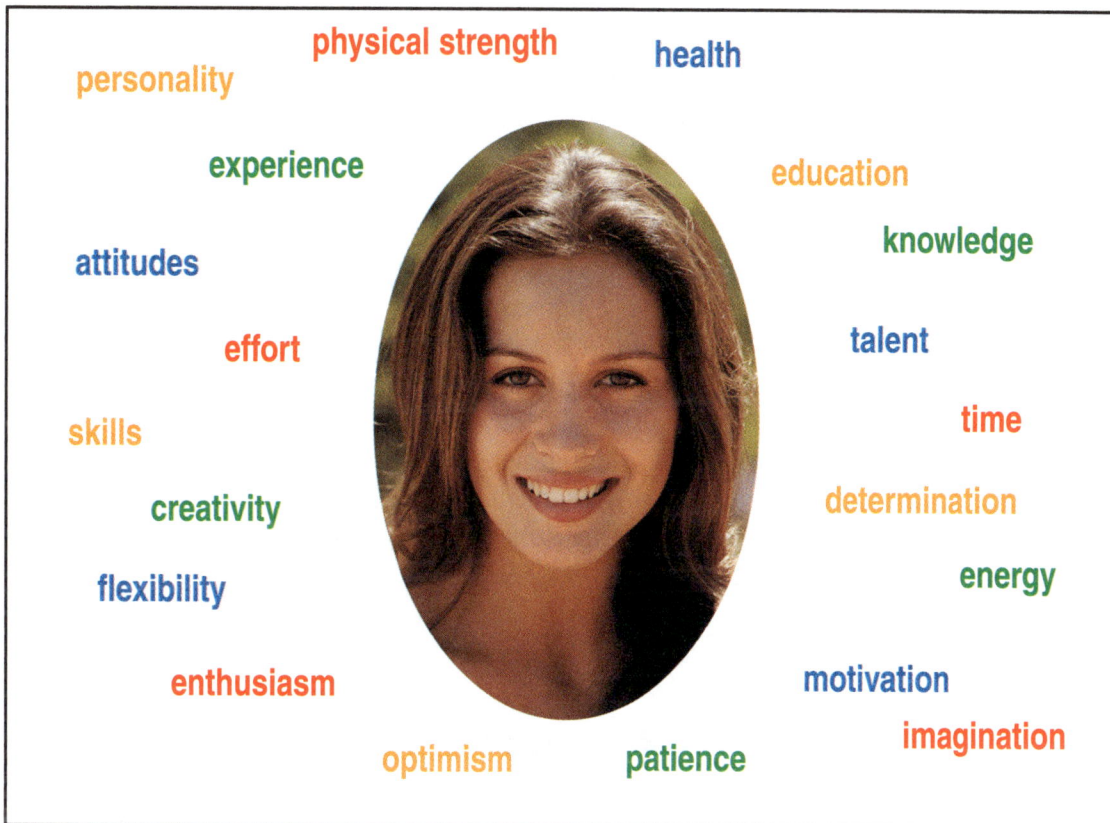

personality
physical strength
health
experience
education
knowledge
attitudes
effort
talent
skills
time
creativity
determination
flexibility
energy
enthusiasm
motivation
imagination
optimism
patience

3-1 Think about your human resources—what strengths within you can you use to reach your goals? What help can others offer?

Determination means committing to hold firmly to the plan you've chosen. It means doing what it takes to reach your goals. You may rely on determination to help you get up, dressed, and off to school no matter how tired you are. This trait will help you focus when you start to get off track. It may take determination to meet all your baby's needs. Being committed to your child will bring you home when you'd like to be out with friends. It is determination that makes difficult tasks possible.

Flexibility means being ready and able to adapt to change. This trait will help you deal with new or unplanned situations. People who are flexible can adjust to change. They find ways to handle tough times and improve their circumstances. When a sudden change forces you to cancel your plans, flexibility can help you find useful ways to spend your time. It will also help you see new options. Being flexible makes difficult tasks a little easier.

Material Resources

Material resources are all those objects you own or can use. The most common material resource is money. With money, you can pay for the goods and services you need. If your goal is to go to college, you will need the money for tuition, fees, books, and supplies. You might work to save this money or apply for grants and loans. You could also ask the public aid office what help might be available.

Other objects and equipment are material resources, too. An example is a car or bicycle that can take you where you need to go. The newspaper, telephone, and Internet can also be resources. You can use these tools to find answers to questions you have. For more examples, see Figure 3-2. Which ones do you have? How might you use some of these resources?

Community Resources

A third type is community resources. These are the facilities and services that are available to you because you live in the community. Community resources include libraries, schools, clinics, and police departments.

Material Resources

❖ **Financial**—money, food stamps, credit, Medicaid, TANF, child support

❖ **Community facilities and services**—schools, libraries, hospitals, health departments, parks, public transportation, fire and police protection, houses of worship, community centers, and shelters

❖ **Tools and equipment**—telephone, home appliances, television, radio, computer, Internet, sewing machine, car, bicycle, newspapers, books, magazines, and supplies

❖ **Business and industry**—the marketplace of goods and services, jobs, training programs factories, communications, and entertainment

❖ **Government facilities and services**—government agencies that provide services and information, such as the Social Security Administration, public aid programs, education, Department of Health and Human Services, and job training programs

3-2 If you look hard enough, you will find that a host of material resources is available to you.

Your town or city may also run programs for pregnant and parenting teens. These can be very helpful. Find out what resources your area offers. Use these resources wisely to help you reach your goals.

Managing Your Resources

Resources are always limited. They never come in an endless supply. If you use a given resource for one purpose, it will not be available for something else. When you spend time talking on the phone, you can't use this same time for studying. While resources are limited, your needs are not. Meeting your needs is an ongoing process. If you parent, you must meet your baby's needs, too. You must plan carefully. By managing your resources, you can get the most benefit from them.

Resources can often work together. For instance, you can combine your time and experience to shop carefully and stretch your dollars. You could use your energy and talent to find a job that will earn more money. Friends and family are often resources, too. Suppose an aunt offers to babysit and a friend offers to drive you to school each day. With their help, it would be easier for you to finish school. Look around. You may find resources you never noticed before.

Managing your resources means putting them to their best use to help you meet your goals. To do this, you should take a careful look at your needs and goals. Then decide how you can use your resources to meet these needs and goals. You can use the following questions to guide you:

- What goals should I set? What do I want to obtain or achieve? What do I value most? (Examples are a healthy baby, food, shelter, clothes, a high school diploma, and finding a job. Set goals related to your values.)
- What stands between me and my goals? What must I overcome? (Examples are lack of money, child care, or transportation; health problems, and incomplete education—anything that makes it harder to meet your goals. For each goal, list the obstacles that stand in your way. Try to find ways to overcome these hurdles.)
- What resources can I use to overcome these obstacles and reach my goals? (Examples are time, money, experience, education, help from your partner or family, and public aid. Put all your resources to work for you.)

You may wish to write the answers to these questions on a piece of paper. Figure 3-3 lists goals, obstacles, and resources many pregnant and parenting teens have. Consider these as they relate to your situation. You can create a similar chart of your own. Use this chart to plan how you will use your resources to reach your most important goals.

From time to time, evaluate your progress toward your goals. This will keep you on track. It will also help you adjust your plans as needed to reach the goals you have set. Evaluating can help you make the best use of your resources to meet your goals. Use the questions listed in Figure 3-4 to help you evaluate your plans, actions, and results.

Managing Resources

Common Goals	Possible Obstacles	Possible Resources
To obtain crib, car seat, clothes, and other necessary equipment for my baby	❖ cost of equipment ❖ lack of experience in choosing baby things ❖ no knowledge of what to buy or where to start	❖ financial help from family, partner, or TANF ❖ resale shops or baby equipment exchanges ❖ advice from parents, counselors, pediatrician, and other moms ❖ parenting brochures, books, and magazines; reputable Web sites
To complete high school, GED, or job-training program	❖ cost of books, clothes, child care, and transportation ❖ inadequate child care ❖ feeling out of place ❖ exhaustion from pregnancy and parenting ❖ discouragement	❖ public aid and social service programs for pregnant and parenting ❖ alternative schools or school programs that offer child care ❖ support from family and friends ❖ dedicated caseworkers, teachers, and counselors ❖ legislation guaranteeing your rights to education
To get a good job	❖ lack of job skills and experience ❖ not knowing how to create a resume or present self to a potential employer ❖ not knowing how to find work, apply for a job, and interview ❖ not knowing what it takes to keep a job and do it well ❖ no high school diploma ❖ lack of child care or cost of child care ❖ lack of confidence ❖ being unaware of job openings ❖ no clothes for work or interviews	❖ job training programs ❖ job counseling ❖ employment office ❖ school or public library; Internet ❖ GED testing or alternative school programs ❖ family help with child care or child care assistance through TANF ❖ support from family, counselors, and teachers ❖ practice and mock interviews ❖ a mentor at school or youth center ❖ recommendation from teachers, counselors, and former employers ❖ clothing program for those entering the workforce for the first time

3-3 As you manage your resources, you may find it helpful to create a chart similar to this. Write your goals, the obstacles you face, and the resources you have that might help you.

Evaluating Your Progress

The Plan

- ❖ What are your goals?
- ❖ Are these goals realistic, specific, and measurable?
- ❖ What obstacles stand in your way?
- ❖ Do you have a workable plan for overcoming these obstacles?
- ❖ What resources do you need?
- ❖ Are these resources available to you?
- ❖ What other resources do you have that could be helpful?
- ❖ Are your goals worth the effort and resources you must use to attain them?

Your Actions

- ❖ How well is your plan working?
- ❖ Are you making progress toward your goals?
- ❖ Are you making the best use of your resources?
- ❖ Does the way you use resources reflect your priorities?
- ❖ Can you improve your planning and follow-through?
- ❖ Have unexpected events created a need to change your plans?

The Results

- ❖ Did you reach your goals?
- ❖ Was reaching your goals worth the effort and resources it took?
- ❖ Are you satisfied with the results?
- ❖ What were the key factors in your reaching (or failing to reach) your goals?
- ❖ How can you improve your planning in the future?

As you think through these questions, look for ways to improve your results and future planning. You will need to adjust your plan as circumstances change.

3-4 Use these questions to help you evaluate your progress in managing your resources.

Money Management

To get the most benefit from your money, you need to have a plan. This plan will reflect the goals you have set and the steps you will take to reach them. It should guide how you use your money. This plan is called a budget. A simple budget will help you stretch your money and avoid financial problems. To manage your money, it is best to follow six key steps.

Step One: Set Financial Goals.

The amount of money you have is limited. This means you must choose carefully how you will spend it. To use your money to its fullest advantage, you need to set goals. Setting goals means you decide what your priorities will be. Then you can form a plan for your spending and saving that will reflect these priorities.

Time is a major element in the goals you set. For each goal, think about how long it will take you to reach it. Some goals must be met right away. These are immediate goals. Other goals are short-term goals. These are goals you want to meet within a few months. A mid-term goal can be reached in several months or even a year. Long-term goals take more than a year to reach. Often, they might take as long as three or more years to complete.

What do you hope to achieve with the money you have? What do you need and what can you afford? Right now, an immediate goal may be providing for your baby with whatever help you can find. A mid-term goal may be to finish high school. Your long-term goal may be to provide for both of you on your own—without help from your family or public aid. You may do this by finding a full-time job after high school.

Decide what you want to accomplish most now and in the future. List 5 to 10 of your important financial goals. Rank them from most to least important. Set a time frame in which you will achieve each. See Figure 3-5. Plan to reach your most important and immediate goal first, but always keep your long-term goals in mind. Focusing on your future goals can help you control your spending.

Step Two: Estimate Income and Resources.

In this step, you determine what you have to work with in meeting your expenses and reaching your goals. First, you must figure your total monthly income. If you work, the money you earn from your job is income. Cash assistance from the Temporary Assistance for Needy Families (TANF) Bureau is

Setting Financial Goals

Financial Goals	When Wanted	Estimated Cost	Amount I Have	Amount I Need
Short-Term Goals (within six months)				
1. _____	1. _____	1. _____	1. _____	1. _____
2. _____	2. _____	2. _____	2. _____	2. _____
3. _____	3. _____	3. _____	3. _____	3. _____
Mid-Term Goals (six months to a year)				
1. _____	1. _____	1. _____	1. _____	1. _____
2. _____	2. _____	2. _____	2. _____	2. _____
3. _____	3. _____	3. _____	3. _____	3. _____
Long-Term Goals (one to five years)				
1. _____	1. _____	1. _____	1. _____	1. _____
2. _____	2. _____	2. _____	2. _____	2. _____
3. _____	3. _____	3. _____	3. _____	3. _____

3-5 You may want to create a chart such as this one to help you set financial goals. Being clear about what's important to you will help you reach these goals.

income, too. If you receive child support regularly, you can also count this. However, don't count child support as income if you don't receive the full amount each month.

Besides income, there are other related resources to keep in mind. If you can use a resource in place of money, this will give you more money for other purposes. This can help you stretch your money farther. What noncash benefits do you receive from the government? For instance, if you get food stamps and Medicaid, you will spend much less on food and health care. You may receive other free or low-cost services, too. An example is living with your family and having relatives help with child care.

List all the sources of income and resources you can rely on in the months ahead. Next to each source of income, write the amount you can expect from this source monthly. For money from a job, give the net pay, or the amount of your check after taxes and deductions. See Figure 3-6 for a sample chart you can use.

Step Three: Estimate Expenses.

Expenses are your living costs. They include everything you buy and all the bills you must pay. You need to pay your expenses with the income you receive. To do this, it will be necessary to keep track

Estimating Income

Week or Month of _____			
Income Source	Estimated Income	Actual Income	Comments
Job	$	$	
TANF	$	$	
Family	$	$	
Partner	$	$	
Child Support	$	$	
Other	$	$	
Totals	**$**	**$**	

3-6 Estimating your income will reveal how much money you have to work with each budget period.

of your expenses for a period of time. Then you will need to adjust your spending to fit your income.

When you move out on your own, you'll have many new expenses. Some of these are rent, utilities, and insurance. Setting up and running a home costs money. You will also need to pay for food, health care, transportation, clothes, and personal supplies. This doesn't even include entertainment or other costs.

Having a baby will also bring new expenses you may never have considered. These will include medical bills; child care; diapers; baby clothes, supplies, and food; baby equipment and toys. Write a list of the items you will need. Include the estimated costs of each item. Figure these expenses into your budget.

There are three main ways to think about your expenses. You can separate needs from wants, routine from occasional spending, and fixed from flexible expenses. When you think about your expenses in these ways, it becomes easier to manage your money.

Needs Versus Wants

The term needs describes items and services you must have. You and your baby need shelter, food, and basic clothing. Heating, cooling, water, electricity, and health care cost money, too. These are expenses you cannot eliminate. You can, however, shop wisely in these areas and keep your costs to a minimum.

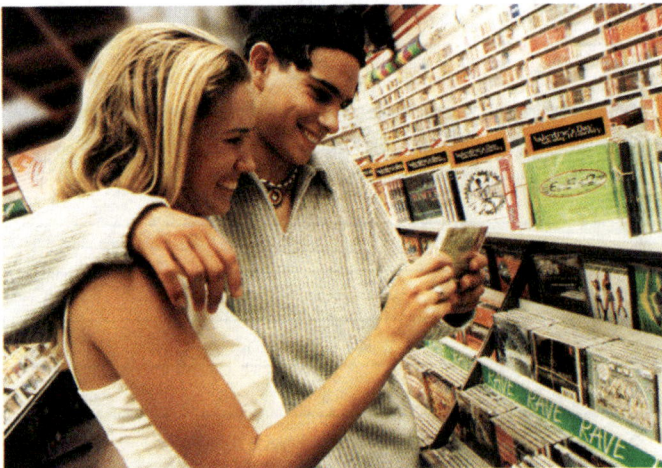

Wants are items and services you would like but can live without. Examples are extra clothing, toys, movies, jewelry, and makeup. Wants are things you should only buy if you can afford them. See Figure 3-7. Meet your needs before spending money on these items.

3-7 Buying CDs is fun, but not necessary for survival. Wait to buy want items until all your important needs are met.

No two people will come up with the same need and want list. Try to divide your expenses into <u>need</u> and <u>want</u> categories as you see them. In managing money, it will be important to buy the items on your need list before those on the want list.

Routine Versus Occasional Spending

Part of managing your money is keeping your spending under control. You must also be ready to meet expenses. Your first question should be when must the expense be paid. Routine expenses are those that must be paid on a regular basis. You can think of these as everyday costs. Some arise weekly or monthly, such as rent or transportation. Others, such as food, are less regular but still occur often. Routine expenses for your baby are diapers, health checkups, and child care. As you create a budget, don't forget to include your routine expenses.

You must also pay some expenses that are less predictable. Occasional expenses are costs that arise from time to time. Some of these are one-time costs, such as a crib. Once you have paid these costs, they do not occur again. Others are recurring costs. These costs may occur once or twice a year. Examples are taxes, insurance, and gifts. Don't forget to plan ahead for occasional and one-time expenses. See Figure 3-8. It is important to save in advance so you can pay these costs when they arise.

Estimating Occasional and One-Time Expenses for the Coming Year

Expense	Need By	Estimated	Actual
Baby equipment		$	$
Furniture		$	$
Home appliances		$	$
Gifts		$	$
Taxes		$	$
Insurance		$	$
Other		$	$
	Totals	$	$

3-8 No one wants to be surprised by unexpected expenses. It's best to plan ahead for the occasional and one-time expenses you will face.

Fixed Versus Flexible Expenses

You can also divide your expenses into the groups <u>fixed</u> and <u>flexible</u>. See Figure 3-9. A fixed expense comes due at a set time each month or year. Examples are rent, utility bills, insurance, and taxes. Some, such as rent, are a set amount every month or year.

Estimating Fixed and Flexible Expenses

Week or Month of _____			
Flexible Expenses	**Estimated**	**Actual**	**Comments**
Utilities (electric, gas, water, trash, phone, cable)	$	$	
Food	$	$	
Household supplies	$	$	
Baby supplies	$	$	
Personal supplies	$	$	
Child care	$	$	
Transportation	$	$	
Health care	$	$	
Savings	$	$	
Entertainment	$	$	
Gifts	$	$	
Other	$	$	
Total - Flexible Expenses			
Fixed Expenses			
Rent or mortgage	$	$	
Car payment	$	$	
Insurance	$	$	
Taxes	$	$	
Tuition	$	$	
Other	$	$	
Total - Fixed Expenses	$	$	
Total–All Expenses (Fixed and Flexible)	$	$	

3-9 Fixed expenses are often the same from one budget period to the next. Flexible expenses are more likely to vary.

Others, such as your electric bill, will vary somewhat each time. Plan ahead for fixed expenses. Pay them on time when they come due. This will build your reputation as a responsible person. It will also help you avoid many financial problems.

A flexible expense offers some leeway about when you pay for it. Food, household supplies, clothing, and grooming items are a few examples. You may be able to decide when you buy these things and how much you will pay. You may be able to delay buying these items for a short time when you are short of cash. If a flexible expense won't wait, you may be able to buy it in a smaller amount until you have more money. For instance, you might buy half a gallon of milk instead of a full gallon until you get paid. This might get you by for a few days.

Step Four: Create a Budget.

A budget is a written plan. It lets you handle your spending and savings in a businesslike manner. A budget will help you keep track of your money. It will direct your income to your most vital expenses. Figure 3-10 shows one way to set up a trial budget. You can use this form or develop a similar plan that will work for you.

You may wonder how long your budget period should be. Set your budget period to match the times when you receive money. If this is only once a month, try a monthly budget. With weekly or biweekly (every two weeks) income, a shorter budget period may work better.

The main idea of a budget is to balance your income and expenses. You cannot spend more money than you have. You must make your resources stretch to meet your needs. If money is left over, put some into savings and use the rest on some of your most important wants.

When you can, set aside some money each budget period for savings. This will help you build a cushion against unexpected expenses and emergencies. Otherwise, these sudden expenses can destroy your budget. An emergency can create financial hardship.

Trial Budget		
Week or Month of _____	Planned	Actual
Income		
Job	$	$
TANF	$	$
Family	$	$
Partner	$	$
Child support	$	$
Other	$	$
Total Income	$	$
Expenses		
Fixed Expenses	$	$
Flexible Expenses	$	$
Savings for one-time and	$	$
occasional expenses	$	$
Total Expenses	$	$
Balance	$	$

3-10 You can use a form like this one to create a trial budget. Refer back to your estimates of income and expenses when completing this budget.

If you keep a little cash on hand, you can also afford to take advantage of special sales. You could stock up on diapers when they're on sale. This would save you money over buying them at full price. See Chapter 4 to learn more about saving money as you shop.

At times, though, you may not even have enough money to cover your needs and those of your baby. Many teen parents have this experience at least once in a while. This can be scary. If you plan carefully, you can get through this rough time. Decide which are your most essential needs. (Often these are fixed expenses, such as rent and utility bills. There may be a penalty for paying these bills later than their due dates.) Focus your spending to meet these key needs.

When there's not enough money to cover expenses, look for a way to make changes. You must either bring in more money or spend less. In what ways might you increase your income or resources? Consider the following:

☛ Can you find part-time work?

☛ What can your partner contribute?

☛ Can your family offer a place to live, food, child care, and other help?

☛ Do you qualify for public aid?

☛ Are there local programs that offer support and services for pregnant and parenting teens?

☛ Can you exchange or share child care or baby items with friends or neighbors?

Cutting your expenses may be another option. You may find obvious ways to lower your costs. There may also be creative ways to spend less.

☛ What items that you currently pay for could you do without?

☛ Can you switch to lower-cost brands or services on some items?

☛ Can you postpone purchasing nonessential items?

☛ Can you and someone else purchase a larger size or bulk item together and split it? (For instance, you may be able to buy food in large quantities at a discount. You could divide the food with friends and share the savings.)

☛ Can you locate any resources that would help you reduce or eliminate an expense? (For instance, if you qualify for food stamps, you would reduce or eliminate the expense of groceries.)

Try your best to make your budget balance. Following the steps in Figure 3-11 may help. It may take quite a bit of calculating before you arrive at a balanced budget. Don't give up; you can figure it out. If you get really frustrated, put your papers away for a little while and take a break. When you return, the answer may seem clearer. If you still need help, ask a parent, counselor, or caseworker. This person may have ideas you haven't considered. He or she might

Crunching the Numbers: How to Create a Budget

1. List your total income for the budget period.
2. List your total expenses for the budget period.
3. Subtract your expenses from your income. This amount is your balance.
4. If you have a positive balance, go to step 5. If your balance is negative, it means you don't have enough money to pay your expenses. In this case, adjust the numbers until you find a way to make ends meet. This means raising your income and resources or decreasing your expenses. Work with these amounts until you come out even or ahead at the end of your budget period.
5. If you have a balance, plan ahead for occasional and one-time expenses in the near future. Figure out how many budget periods there are between now and when the expense must be paid. Divide the amount of each expense by the number of budget periods. Insert each amount in your budget under expenses for each of these budget periods. This way you can spread out the cost of these expenses. Adjust as needed to make this work for you.
6. Recopy your budget onto a clean sheet of paper so you can read it easily. Refer to this often and make adjustments when necessary.

3-11 Creating a budget may seem complicated, but it can be done in a few fairly simple steps.

also be able to direct you to someone else who can help. Some consumer agencies offer free or low-cost financial counseling. These agencies are often listed in the Yellow Pages.

Step Five: Follow Your Budget.

In this step, you take action on your budget. Try it out for one or two budget periods. See how the plan you've made will work. If you have trouble some months making income cover expenses, you're not alone. Many people find it hard to come out even or ahead. Don't abandon your budget; adjust it to better fit your situation.

It may help to keep close track of your spending for a few weeks. This will show you where your money goes. Use a small notebook to record your spending. List everything you buy and its cost. This detailed record of spending may surprise you. It can show ways to change spending habits that will free more money for things you really need.

From your record, you may discover ways to reduce spending. Even small amounts of money add up very quickly. For instance, by giving up one $5 fast-food meal each week to eat at home, you would save between $15 and $20 a month. (This figure takes into account that you'd need to spend a few dollars to buy groceries for these at-home meals.) In a year's time, your savings would total at least $200! Think of what you could do with this extra money.

It is important to manage your finances like a business. This can make it possible for you to slowly get ahead and become self-sufficient. See Figure 3-12 for more budgeting tips. Make adjustments to your budget as your goals, income, and expenses change.

Quick Tips for Better Budgeting

❖ Keep it simple.

❖ Prepare for the unexpected.

❖ Write it down.

❖ Keep it all together.

❖ Be specific.

❖ Be disciplined.

❖ Be flexible.

3-12 When working with your financial plans, it may help to keep these tips in mind.

Step Six: Evaluate Your Budget.

Your financial picture can change dramatically almost overnight. It pays to evaluate your money matters every few months. Have you been able to meet your basic financial needs? Can you control your spending? Are you reaching your goals and paying your bills? Do you feel you've made progress? Are you satisfied with how you've managed your money? If the answer to each of these questions is <u>yes</u>, good for you! Otherwise, it's time to look for ways to improve.

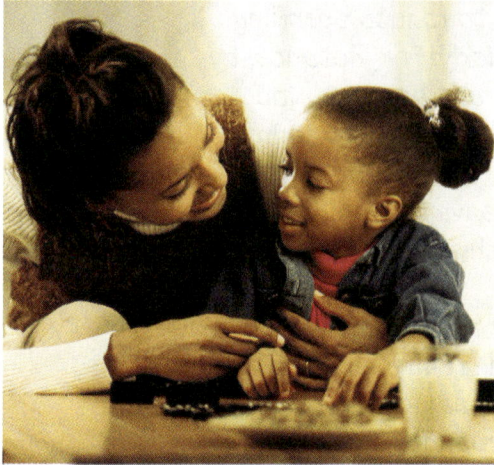

Reviewing your financial plans from time to time is a good idea. In addition, you should rethink your budget again whenever there is a change in your income, resources, expenses, or goals. First, decide if this change means you need to adjust your plans. Next, figure out how you can adjust your budget to meet your changing needs.

Major life changes may require you to redo your budget. At these times, new factors may enter the picture. See Figure 3-13. Decide how to build these factors into your budget. Some examples of major life changes include the following:

3-13 Having a child can mean major changes in your budget!

- ☞ pregnancy or the birth of a child
- ☞ marriage
- ☞ divorce
- ☞ job changes
- ☞ sudden serious illness or disability
- ☞ change in the number of people in your household
- ☞ large change in your income or expenses

When changes cause you to rethink your plan, adjust your budget as needed to keep your finances in control. Evaluating your budget often can help you ensure your money is going to its best use.

Preventing Problems

When it comes to managing money, preventing problems is much easier than fixing them. The effort you use to avoid financial trouble will pay off. Use your resources wisely. This will leave you with more money for your needs and wants. Be cautious when you use credit. The tips on the next page will help you avoid problems with your creditors (the people and companies to whom you owe money).

☛ Create a bill-paying kit. This should include a calendar, pen, envelopes, notepad, stamps, and a folder to store bills waiting to be paid. Being organized will keep you from losing your bills or forgetting when they are due. Staying aware of your bills will help you pay them on time.

☛ Note the date each bill is due before you put it into the folder. Most companies advise you to allow at least five business days for delivery in the mail. Sending in a bill this early helps it arrive on time. This means you can avoid late fees and penalties. Write on your calendar the date each bill is due and when you must mail it. As you refer to your calendar, you can see at a glance when your bills are due.

☛ Read all bills and statements carefully. Sometimes errors are made. If you note any errors, contact the creditor right away. This will help you settle the matter quickly. Ask if you must explain the problem in writing or if a phone call is enough. Keep detailed notes of all contacts you make with the company regarding errors. List the name of the person you talked to as well as the date and time. Write a summary of what was said in the conversation. Attach these notes to your bills for filing.

☛ If financial problems keep you from paying a bill in full on the due date, let the company know. Call <u>before</u> the due date to make payment arrangements. When you call, tell the company how much you can send now and when you can send more. Again, keep notes about each person you talk to regarding your bill. Attach these to a copy of the bill for filing.

  Whatever agreement you make, try as hard as you can to keep your word. This is a responsible approach. It keeps the company willing to work with you. Even if you can only send $10 a month, a company might accept this arrangement. Being faithful in your payments shows your desire to pay.

☛ When you send in a payment, write the date, the amount you paid, and the number of the check or money order you used right on the bill. Maintain a file of past bills so you can refer to them again if needed.

☛ Be careful with your use of credit. If not used properly, this can lead to problems quickly. See Chapter 5 to learn more about credit.

Keeping Records

To stay on top of your finances, you need a workable system of record keeping. For many, this means setting up a filing system to store financial records. You'll need to create a system that works for you. You should save important papers and keep them safely stored. This could be in a drawer, filing cabinet, file box, basket, or notebook. Make sure this place is handy so you can find what you need quickly and easily. File your papers in a way that makes sense to you. See Figure 3-14 for a list of important papers you should keep on file.

You will want to keep a current list of important names, addresses, and phone numbers on file. The list might include health care providers, caseworkers, counselors, and employers. This saves you time by making the numbers easy to find. Update this list from time to time.

Keeping Records: What Should You File?

Some of the important papers you should keep on file include the following:

* check stubs and amounts of cash income from jobs, public aid, and child support
* records and estimated value of noncash resources (food stamps, family support, and Medicaid)
* billing statements and any receipts for bills paid
* information regarding savings or checking accounts you have (account numbers and the names and addresses of the financial institution)
* receipts, owner's manuals, and warranties for items you own
* copies of your income tax records and returns
* credit contracts and records of payments
* personal budget and any other financial records
* employment records

If you are an immigrant, you will also need the following papers:

* Arrival-Departure Record, I-94
* Resident Alien form, I-51 or I-551
* citizenship papers, I-179 or I-197
* proof of citizenship/alien status, if you are applying for public aid or food stamps

3-14 Refer to this list when deciding which items to file and which to throw away.

It's also a good idea to keep up with filing your records away. Otherwise, these papers tend to stack up, making it hard for you to find what you need. Staying organized will help you manage your finances.

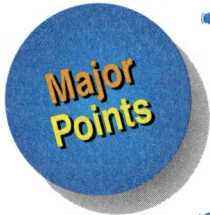

Major Points

☛ Managing your money and resources is particularly challenging when you have little or no money of your own. Your financial well-being will depend on learning to manage well. This takes patience, self-control, and practice.

☛ Many resources are available for your use. It's a good idea to identify the resources you have. This will allow you to use them to their fullest advantage. Each person's list of resources is unique.

☛ To get the most from your resources, you will need to manage them wisely. Sometimes you can combine two or more resources to help you meet a goal. Evaluating your progress should help you make changes when needed.

☛ There are several steps to follow when managing your money. Set clear financial goals. Accurately estimate your income and related resources, as well as all your expenses. Work out a budget to help you control spending and achieve the goals that are important to you. Evaluate your plans from time to time and make the needed adjustments.

☛ It's a good idea to take what steps you can to prevent financial problems. Being a responsible consumer will help you stay out of many financial tangles. When problems arise, try best to solve them as promptly as possible in a businesslike manner.

☛ Part of managing your money is keeping clear and organized records. This lets you find important financial records and documents quickly when you need them. Maintaining a filing system may take some effort, but it will be well worth your time. It will also give you a sense of control.

Chapter 4
Shopping
like a Pro

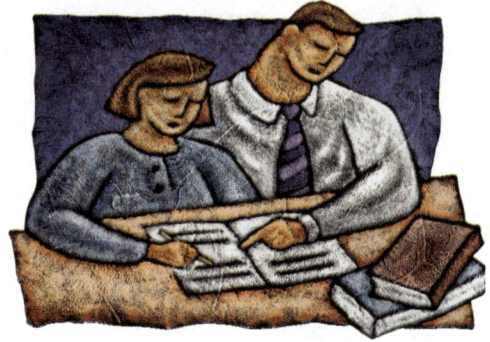

As a consumer, one of your roles is to shop for the goods and services you need and want. Managing your money when shopping is critical. You want to get the most from your money and avoid wasting it. Wise spending choices can help you stretch your dollars.

If you will be parenting, careful use of your money is even more crucial. You will soon have many more expenses than before, as well as the needs of your child to consider. In this chapter, you can learn several skills that will help you become a smart shopper.

Understanding the Marketplace

As a shopper, you choose where to spend your money. There are many places to buy goods and services. The term marketplace refers to all the sellers of goods and services worldwide. Before shopping, you need to know something about sellers as well as the goods and services they provide.

The marketplace offers several types of sellers. You can buy from stores, catalogs, online, or from door-to-door salespeople. Shopping each of these ways has its pros and cons. It's up to you to choose the type of seller that suits you best. You will no doubt shop with more than one seller, depending upon the item or service you need to buy. For instance, you might buy some products from a catalog and others from a neighborhood store.

Neighborhood stores often are convenient. This kind of store is nearby, so you can easily go there to pick up a few items. See Figure 4-1. You may like to shop in a small store where you know the sellers. Buying from these stores also helps build the local economy. Neighborhood stores tend to be small and lack competition, though. This means they often charge higher prices than shopping centers or downtown stores do. Selection in these

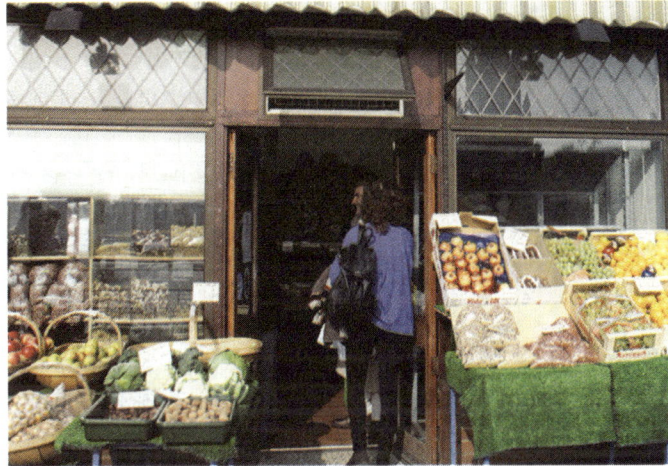

4-1 A neighborhood grocery store may be a good place to pick up a few items quickly.

stores may also be limited. You will often find lower prices and a wider selection at shopping centers or downtown stores.

You can also shop at discount stores or factory outlets. These stores offer lower prices because they often sell discontinued or overstocked items. They buy merchandise at closeout prices and pass the savings to their customers. These stores can offer real bargains.

These stores do not sell the highest quality items. Many of these products will still be good enough to meet your everyday needs. For instance, you don't need top-of-the-line baby clothes that will only be worn a few months. Less expensive clothes will meet your baby's needs just fine. You can put the money you save into buying other items you need.

You may find lower prices at discount stores and factory outlets. You'll lose some of your savings, however, if the store is hard to get to or you must pay transportation costs. Resist the temptation to buy more than you need just because the price is low. If you buy too many items, you'll spend most of your savings.

You may be offered goods from a door-to-door seller. These sellers bring products right into your home. This can be convenient when you know the product so well you don't need to compare it with store products. When a door-to-door seller visits you, ask to see his or her identification and selling permit. Avoid making an impulse buy or being swayed by a clever sales pitch. Buy only items you need. Be sure you fully understand the terms of any contract before you sign it. Keep all papers the seller gives you. Find out how to contact the seller if there's a problem.

The Federal Trade Commission (FTC) passed a law giving consumers the right to cancel most door-to-door purchases within three business days. This lets you get your money back if you have second thoughts. Most states also have a "cooling-off-period" law. Check the law in your state. Don't be afraid to act on your rights.

As the Internet grows more popular, many sellers have set up Web sites where their customers can buy goods and services. You can also buy products from a catalog or mail order seller. Each of these sellers offers a wide variety of goods. This can be a convenient way to shop if you

- are reasonably sure of the quality and important features from the descriptions of the merchandise that are given
- factor the delivery and shipping costs into the price of merchandise
- keep a record of your order including date; total costs; items ordered by item number and style; and the seller's name, address, and phone number
- understand the exchange and return policies and can accept the bother and expense of making returns

Wherever you choose to shop, look for what matters most to you. This list will differ for each shopper. One shopper might value convenience most. Another may care most about finding the lowest prices. Many shoppers search for quality goods and services. They also want fair prices, a wide selection, reliable sales help, a pleasant atmosphere, and honest sales policies. What do you value most? What makes shopping the easiest for you?

Evaluating Sellers

Not all sellers are equal. Some are more reliable, friendly, and honest than others. Choose sellers who care about their customers and the community. These sellers provide helpful sales help and services. They will work hard to get and keep your business. In the long run, you'll be most satisfied by doing business with these sellers. You'll also want to shop in stores where you feel comfortable and your business seems welcome.

Use the questions in Figure 4-2 to be sure you're dealing with an honest and fair seller. If you answer yes to most of these questions, you have likely chosen a good seller. If not, you may want to buy from someone else.

Questions to Ask: Evaluating a Seller

- Is advertising believable and are items available at advertised prices?
- Are salespersons informed and helpful rather than pushy?
- Do you feel you're getting honest and polite answers to questions about products, services, and store policies?
- Are return, exchange, and refund policies fair?
- Does the seller belong to the local Chamber of Commerce or Better Business Bureau?
- Do prices and services compare favorably with other stores and sellers?
- Are people you know satisfied with the store?
- Do you get prompt and courteous attention when you have a problem or complaint?
- Does the management accept responsibility for the actions and behavior of salespeople and other employees?
- Does the seller have a good reputation in the community?

4-2   How do the sellers you use measure up? Is it time to search for a new seller?

Finding Reliable Consumer Information

To make smart choices, you need all the facts about the goods and services you want to buy. One part of shopping is doing the research to find this information. There are many places you can look. A few of these are labels and tags, warranties and manuals,

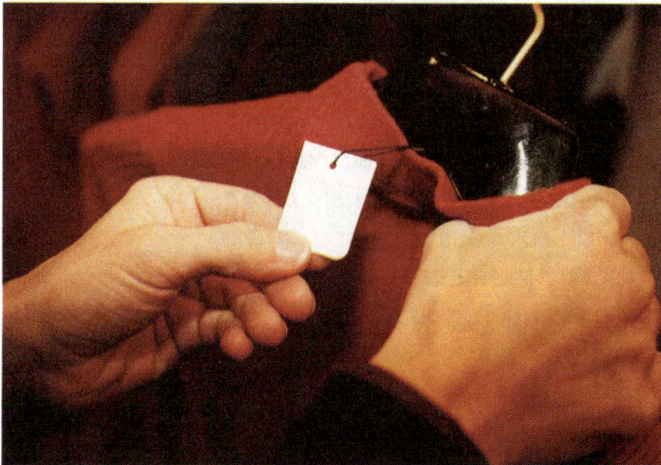

4-3   Smart shoppers always read the clothing labels and tags before making a purchase.

salespeople, and advertisements. You may find other sources that are helpful, too.

Labels and Tags

You will find labels and tags attached to almost all new products you buy. See Figure 4-3. These are a helpful source of product information. Before buying a product, read all the labels and tags to learn more about it.

Laws state what specific information must appear on product labels and tags. All labels must list the brand name of the item, as well as the name and address of its manufacturer. Exactly what else must be on the label varies by product. For instance, a clothing label must state how to care for the garment. It must also tell the fiber content of the fabric. The size of the item appears on the label, too.

Food labels also have many guidelines. All food products must put a list of ingredients on their labels. Most must also carry the Nutrition Facts label. This label gives facts about the nutritional value of the food. See Figure 4-4. It gives the serving size for the food and how many servings are in a container, too.

You may learn other types of information from the label and tags on a product. These may list use and care directions, as well as warnings and cautions about the product. They may describe a product's contents and quality. The label or tag may also tell you

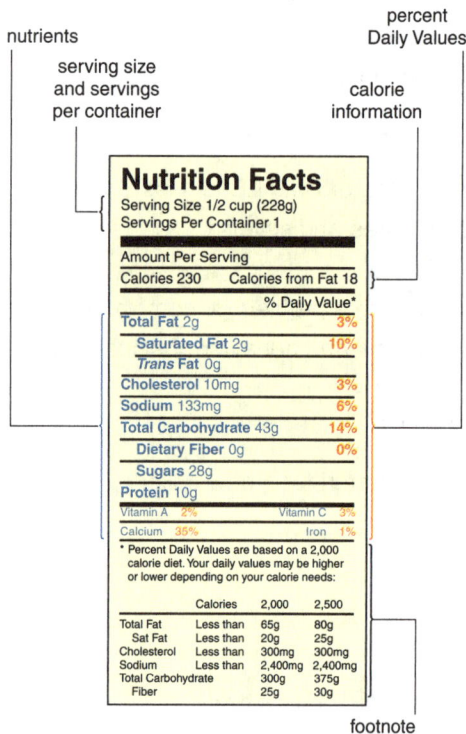

4-4   What can you learn about a food by reading the Nutrition Facts label?

about a product's special features. Many times, you will find a toll-free phone number or Web address on the label or tag. This lets you contact the company to ask more questions about a product.

Written Warranties and Manuals

A warranty is a guarantee from the maker of a product to you, the buyer. The warranty describes what you can expect from a product. It tells what the company will do if the product fails or has defects. Most warranties cover a product for a set period, such as 90 days or 1 year. A written warranty is legally binding. It can be upheld in court if needed. See Figure 4-5 to learn what a written warranty must include.

There are two main types of warranties—full and limited. A full warranty gives the most protection. With this warranty, the company must repair or replace a faulty product or part. They must do so within a reasonable amount of time at no cost to you. If a company tries to repair a product and fails, they must replace the item at no cost to you. A full warranty must last throughout its stated period. This is true even if you give or sell the product to someone else.

A limited warranty gives less protection if a product fails. It may cover repairs but not replacement. You may be asked to return a faulty product to the seller or take it to an approved service

Written Warranties

The law requires a warranty to tell you:

* whether it is full or limited (if it's limited, what the limitations are)

* what it covers—the entire product or only certain parts

* what will be done if the product fails

* what you must do to obtain coverage

* how long coverage lasts

* how to get warranty benefits

4-5 You can learn much about a product by reading the written warranty. How could this information affect your purchase decision?

center for repair. You may have to pay labor costs or handling charges for repairs. A limited warranty may also cover only the first owner of the product. If you sell the product or give it away, the warranty may end.

Some products give a limited warranty on some parts and a full warranty on others. This is often the case with electronic products that have many parts.

Most warranties only cover product defects or failure. They do not repair products damaged by misuse. If you caused the problem, it is likely your warranty won't cover it.

When shopping, you can ask to see the warranty for a product. Read it carefully and ask questions about anything you don't understand. Compare the warranty terms of various brands and models. This may be a factor in your purchase. This is most true when it comes to costly items you expect to use for a long time. The warranty is also important for appliances and equipment that are costly to repair.

The owner's manual or instruction book can also provide key facts about a product. This book will provide instructions on the safe use, care, and maintenance of the product. You will often find the written warranty in this book. Other times it is a separate sheet or booklet. Reading all this information before you buy the product will inform you what you can expect from it.

Salespeople

Salespeople can also be a good source of information. By asking questions, you can learn quite a bit about a product. A helpful salesperson will give you a straight answer about a product or service. This person will know how various brands and models of an item compare. He or she can point out a product's special features. Often, a salesperson can show you how to operate the product. This person may also know when new products are expected and when goods and services will be on sale.

Not all salespeople are good at their jobs or helpful to customers. In fact, some only care about selling more products than anyone else. For this reason, you can't always trust a salesperson's advice. Don't depend solely on what the salesperson says. Seek advice from someone else or do your research. Don't be persuaded to spend more than you had planned. If you feel the least bit pressured or unsure, wait. Come back to the store another time to make your purchase. This will give you some time to make up your mind.

Treat salespeople with respect and kindness. In return, they will often give you better service and more information. You will be more likely to receive the help you need. When you find a helpful salesperson, shop with this person again. Over time, you can build a solid business relationship with him or her. You will feel you can trust this salesperson's advice.

Advertising

Companies use advertising as a tool to help them sell goods and services. An advertisement, or ad, is a message that promotes goods or services. The company pays for this ad. Many ads appear in magazines and newspapers. See Figure 4-6. They can also be found online and on billboards and signs. Ads that are broadcast on TV or radio are often called commercials.

The main purpose of an ad or commercial is to sell a product or service. You can also learn a lot from commercials. Some of this information can help you make shopping choices. Often ads include facts about the following:

- ☛ prices
- ☛ features
- ☛ brands

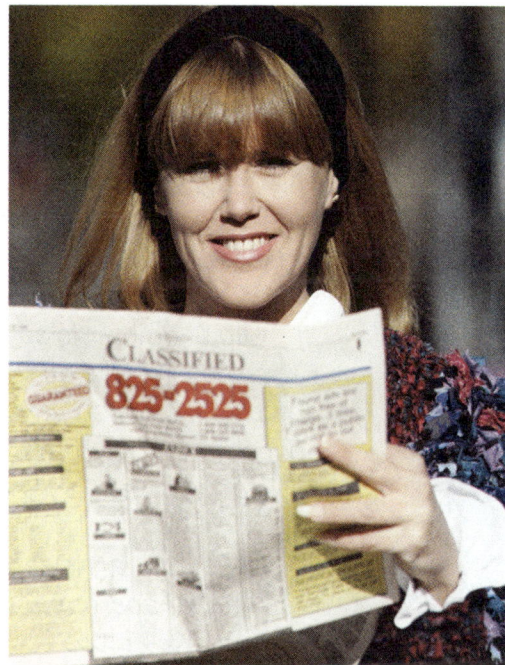

4-6 Most newspapers contain store ads as well as a classified advertising section. You can gain product information by reading these.

- ☞ model numbers
- ☞ services
- ☞ deliveries
- ☞ new products
- ☞ product descriptions
- ☞ special offers
- ☞ names of sellers who carry the product

To make the best use of advertising, look for the facts you need to make a wise choice. Don't be influenced by the opinions stated in the ad or the flashy way in which the product is promoted. Some ads make exaggerated claims. If an advertising claim seems too good to be true, it probably is. Also avoid letting ads sway you to buy goods and services you don't need.

Other Sources of Consumer Information

There are many other ways to learn about products and services. First, you can read consumer articles in newspapers and magazines. These reports should focus on the facts when comparing products. An example is <u>Consumer Reports</u> magazine. This magazine doesn't sell advertising space. For this reason, its reports are less likely to be biased. Many shoppers trust this magazine as a place to seek information.

Clip useful articles from the magazines or newspapers you own. Keep these on file so you can find them easily later. What if you don't subscribe to any papers or magazines? Read them at your school or public library. Be sure to photocopy, rather than clip, articles you want to keep.

Consumer articles also appear on the Internet. You can read many newspapers and magazines online. It's also possible to visit company Web sites to research products. If you can get online, you may find this is a great research tool. It's often a fast and easy way to find up-to-date information.

You can also turn to government publications for the facts you need. The Consumer Information Center (CIC) in Pueblo, Colorado, offers consumer brochures. You can get most at little or no cost. Some brochures list factors to think about as you make buying choices. Others can tell you about the laws related to a product or service. You can contact this office to learn more.

Suppose someone you know has already made the purchase you're considering. Ask this person about it. He or she can tell you what was learned in the shopping process. This may include the following:

- which stores carry the item or provide the service
- what prices these stores charge
- reasons for choosing the goods or services he or she did
- whether the person feels pleased with the purchase now

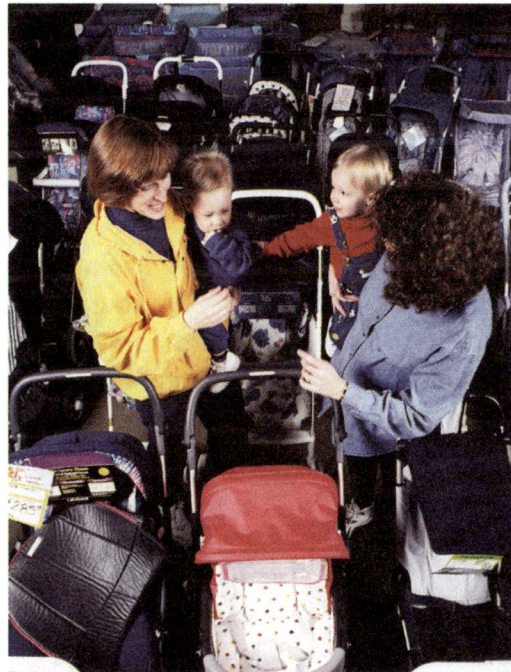

4-7 When shopping for baby items, you might take a friend with you who has already made the same purchase decisions.

You may wonder how accurate this information is. This will depend on who is giving it. Use your judgment when choosing whether to trust this person's advice. If this is a person you trust, you might even take him or her shopping with you. See Figure 4-7.

As you can see, you have many options in finding consumer information. Be sure to learn all you can before making a major purchase. Being informed makes it more likely you will be pleased with your choice. It will also ensure you make the best use of your shopping dollars.

Developing Shopping Skills

To be a smart shopper, you'll need to develop certain skills. Some shopping skills apply to almost any buying decision. Others apply to the purchase of specific goods, such as food or clothing. Buying services and shopping at sales also take some special skills. Learning these skills may take some practice, but it will be well worth your time.

General Shopping Skills

General shopping skills are those that apply to almost every purchase you make. These skills can help you make the best use of your shopping dollars. Use the following guidelines to help you build general shopping skills:

- Exercise self-control and avoid impulse buys. Having self-control means being able to monitor your own actions and make appropriate choices. Self-control helps you stick to your budget. It can also help you avoid impulse buys. These are buys made on the spur of the moment with little thought. Impulse buys can quickly lead you to overspend.
- Decide beforehand what you will buy and how much you can afford to spend. Form a plan and stick to it. If you need to buy more than one item, write a list and follow it. Don't be tempted to pick up other items or go over your spending limit.
- Compare before you buy. Look at many brands and models of the product you want to buy. Review the safety and performance features of each. Also ask about the delivery and installation fees, warranty terms, and the policies of each seller. Lastly, compare prices by brand, model, and store. The price may vary greatly among brands or models. Two stores may even charge different prices for the exact same item.
- Consider the value of your time and energy as you shop. Shopping at discount stores can save you money but may cost you a lot of time and energy. Subtract from your savings the cost of transportation to and from distant stores. Combine your shopping trips to save time, energy, and money. Try to make one trip to a store rather than many.
- Deal fairly and honestly with others when you shop. See Figure 4-8 for tips on treating others with fairness and courtesy. You'll get better service and more respect if you follow these tips. Shopping is also more pleasant when you're kind to other shoppers.

Shopping Fairness Guide

With Other Shoppers	With Businesses	With Salespeople	With Professionals
❖ Wait your turn when several shoppers want help at the same time.	❖ Let merchants and companies know what you like or dislike about their products, services, and policies.	❖ Be respectful and polite, even when there's a problem.	❖ Be on time for appointments.
❖ Avoid pushing, shoving, and raising your voice.	❖ Make necessary returns and exchanges promptly.	❖ Avoid shopping just before closing time.	❖ Call in advance if you must be late or cancel an appointment.
❖ Watch your children and shopping cart carefully.	❖ Be businesslike when handling problems and making complaints.	❖ Handle the merchandise with care and return it to its proper place.	❖ Pay promptly unless you've made credit arrangements.
❖ Avoid blocking the aisles. Other shoppers need to get through.	❖ Avoid damaging merchandise or making unfair returns or exchanges.	❖ If goods are damaged or broken, tell the salesperson.	❖ Except in an emergency, call during office hours. When possible, call in advance to arrange an appointment.
❖ Be courteous. Respect the needs and belongings of other shoppers.	❖ Respect the property of the business facility.	❖ Thank helpful salespeople and ask for their help when you go to the store again.	❖ Respect the expertise of the professionals who serve you. Cooperate with them.

4-8 Follow these tips to become a fair and courteous shopper.

☞ Report unfair or dishonest business practices. If you feel you've been treated unfairly, don't keep quiet about it. Tell the proper authorities. This will help put dishonest sellers out of business or make them change their practices. Figure 4-9 suggests whom to contact when problems occur.

Reporting Consumer Problems

If you have serious problems with a seller, try contacting

❖ Chamber of Commerce

❖ Better Business Bureau

❖ Federal Trade Commission

❖ Local or state consumer protection agencies

❖ State Attorney General's office

4-9 If a seller refuses to correct a consumer problem to your satisfaction, contact one of these agencies for help.

Buying Goods

When you're buying goods, general shopping skills will come in handy. You'll also need to develop some specific skills related to buying goods. You may face many choices each time you buy a product. Sometimes this can make it difficult to decide what you need and want. When you buy goods, take care to do the following:

- Inspect before you buy. Look products over carefully before you buy them. Be sure to choose an item that is well made and in good condition. For instance, when buying clothes, you should try them on to check quality, fit, size, and color. Inspecting products matters most when returns are not allowed.

- Read labels, tags, instruction manuals, and warranties. Look for useful information about the products you want to buy. Find out how the product was made, how to use and care for it, and how to get warranty service if needed. What you learn may affect your decision to buy or not to buy.

- Request demonstrations. Ask to see how appliances and equipment operate. A salesperson may be able to show you how the product works. Check the controls to make sure you know how they work. Before you buy, it's good to know how to use the product and feel sure you can do it with ease.

☞ Decide what characteristics and features are important to you. Many products offer special features and frills. Which of these do you need and want? If a feature affects how you will use the product, you may decide it's worth the cost. How much does this feature raise the price of the product? What extra features can you afford?

☞ Compare new with used products. Purchasing used rather than new goods can save you a lot of money. For example, you can furnish a home with used furniture at a fraction of the cost you would pay for new. When considering a purchase, decide whether used items would be acceptable for your needs.

There are some items you will want to buy new. Most others you can buy used. Compare the costs of new products with used. How much would you save by buying used? Places to buy used goods include resale stores, auctions, garage sales, and military surplus stores. You can also find used items advertised in the newspaper. Ask the seller whether the used items you buy come with a warranty.

Buying Food

Food is a major cost—one you'll have to pay over and over again. The foods you choose will also directly affect your health and fitness. Poor eating can make you feel run down and tired. It can also lead to health problems. By eating well, you will feel better and be in better health. This is why smart food shopping is important. It's good for your budget and well-being.

Buy as much nutritious food as you can with the money you have. To do this you must plan well-balanced, healthful meals and snacks. If you're like most people, you need a little help in knowing which types of food you need and how much of each type to eat. You can use two important guides—MyPyramid and the Dietary Guidelines for Americans—as you plan your menus.

MyPyramid is a personalized food system that helps you plan a healthier diet. It also promotes physical activity. See 4-10. You can access it at www.mypyramid.gov.

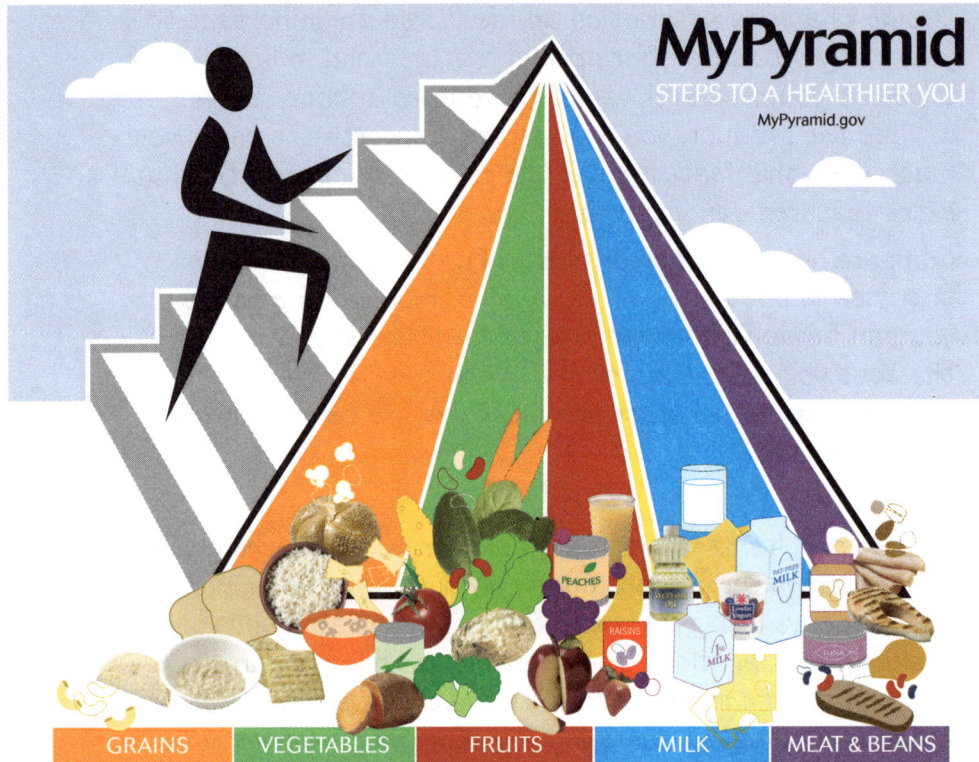

MyPyramid
STEPS TO A HEALTHIER YOU
MyPyramid.gov

GRAINS VEGETABLES FRUITS MILK MEAT & BEANS

4-10 For your good health and your baby's, you need to eat foods from each group every day.

The Dietary Guidelines for Americans are suggestions on healthful eating habits. They were created by the U.S. Department of Agriculture (USDA) and the U.S. Department of Health and Human Services. If you follow the Dietary Guidelines, you can plan more nutritious meals and snacks. See Figure 4-11.

You can also get the most from your food dollars if you remember to do the following:

☞ Check food pages and ads in local papers for prices, specials, and menu ideas. Clip coupons to lower the cost of products you would normally buy. To further cut costs, plan your weekly meals around seasonal foods and sale items.

☞ Use basic cookbooks and food magazines to find menu ideas and recipes. Outline meal, snack, and leftover plans for the week. Buy the items you need to fit these plans.

Dietary Guidelines for Americans
Finding Your Way to a Healthier You

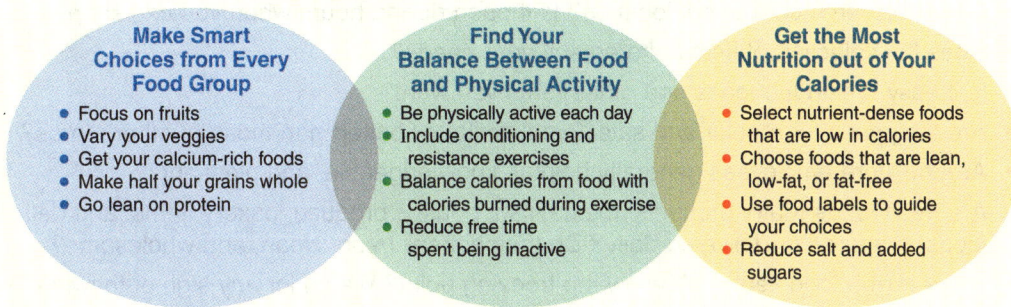

Make Smart Choices from Every Food Group
- Focus on fruits
- Vary your veggies
- Get your calcium-rich foods
- Make half your grains whole
- Go lean on protein

Find Your Balance Between Food and Physical Activity
- Be physically active each day
- Include conditioning and resistance exercises
- Balance calories from food with calories burned during exercise
- Reduce free time spent being inactive

Get the Most Nutrition out of Your Calories
- Select nutrient-dense foods that are low in calories
- Choose foods that are lean, low-fat, or fat-free
- Use food labels to guide your choices
- Reduce salt and added sugars

4-11 Following the Dietary Guidelines for Americans can help you improve your eating habits and your overall health.

☞ Shop only as often as you must, perhaps once a week. The less often you're in the store, the fewer chances you have to overspend. Between shopping trips, keep an ongoing list. Add items to it as you run low. Include foods for planned meals and sale items you want to buy.

☞ Stick to your list when shopping. Avoid food shopping when you're hungry. Your hunger could tempt you to stray from your list.

☞ Try store brands or generic items. Generic products come in plain packages without brand names, which means low packaging costs. Both generic and store-brand products cost much less than national-brand products. The quality of these products may be slightly lower, though. Try generic or store brand foods to discover which ones you like. The savings will be well worth it.

☞ Choose supermarkets and food stores with care. The service, prices, and quality of products will vary depending on where you shop. See Figure 4-12.

☞ Compare food labels to find the most nutritious products. This can make you aware of the content of the foods you're eating. Choose the product that will provide the most nutrients.

☞ Pay attention to dates on food packages. The later the date, the fresher the product will be. Some dates say sell by, while others say use by. A sell-by date tells when the grocer should pull the item from the shelf. A use-by date tells when

Choosing a Place to Buy Food

❖ Is the store clean and well-maintained?

❖ Is the store in a convenient location? Is it open during hours when you can shop?

❖ Does the selection of items offered suit your needs?

❖ Is it easy to find the foods and other items you want?

❖ Are the prices for regular and sale items similar or better than those of other stores?

❖ Are the store employees generally helpful, knowledgeable, and pleasant?

❖ Are fresh foods (dairy products, meats, fish, poultry, produce, bakery items, and deli foods) prepared or delivered daily? Do they appear fresh, clean, and wholesome?

❖ Is the frozen food kept well below the freezing point? Watch for any sign of thawing in the frozen food section. Avoid partially-thawed foods.

❖ Does the store have the departments you want or need, such as deli and pharmacy?

❖ Does the store offer check cashing, coupon exchanges, unit pricing, open dating, nutrition information, and other services you want or need?

❖ Does the store have fair policies, such as honest advertising, rain checks for specials that run out, and replacements or refunds for purchases that are not satisfactory?

❖ Is the overall atmosphere of the store acceptable to you?

4-12 Consider the answers to these questions as you choose places to shop for food.

you should use the food for the best taste and quality. Do not buy food marked with a sell-by date that has passed.

☛ Compare unit prices. The unit price is the price of an item per unit, weight, or measure. You can use this price to compare cost by brand or size of container. The unit price is often given on a label attached to the store shelf beneath the item. See Figure 4-13. If no unit price is given, you can estimate the unit cost in your head or figure it with a calculator.

Unit Pricing

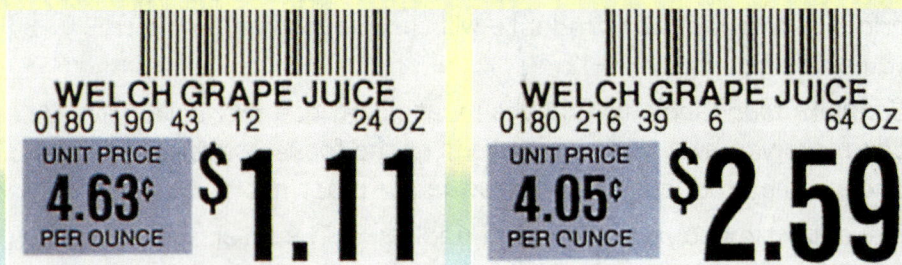

WELCH GRAPE JUICE
0180 190 43   12   24 OZ
UNIT PRICE 4.63¢ PER OUNCE $1.11

WELCH GRAPE JUICE
0180 216 39   6   64 OZ
UNIT PRICE 4.05¢ PER OUNCE $2.59

4-13 Look at the unit prices given for two containers of grape juice that are the same brand but different sizes. Which is a better value?

Buying Clothing

It takes some practice to get the most for your money when buying clothes. Whether you're shopping for you or your baby, it pays to plan before you buy. This helps you get the items you'll need most. Before shopping, ask yourself the following questions:

- ☛ What do my child and I already have?
- ☛ What do we need?
- ☛ What can I afford to spend on clothing now?

The type of clothing you need depends on your lifestyle. See Figure 4-14. What kind of clothes do you need for school? Many teens wear mostly T-shirts and jeans, while some must wear school uniforms. This will depend on your school's dress code. If you work, what type of work clothes are you expected to wear? Do you have to wear dress clothes or is there a uniform? What types of other activities and special occasions do you have? What kind of clothes do you need for these?

If you're a teen parent, buying yourself clothes may be a matter of need rather than want. Your extra money is limited, and you must buy clothes for your child, too. Young children quickly outgrow their clothes and must get larger ones.

4-14 For most teens, jeans fit their lifestyle and needs. What types of clothing do you need?

After you have assessed your clothing needs, think about what you already have. Write a list of the clothing items you need. Rank the items on your list from most to least important. Before you shop, decide how much you can afford to spend based on your budget.

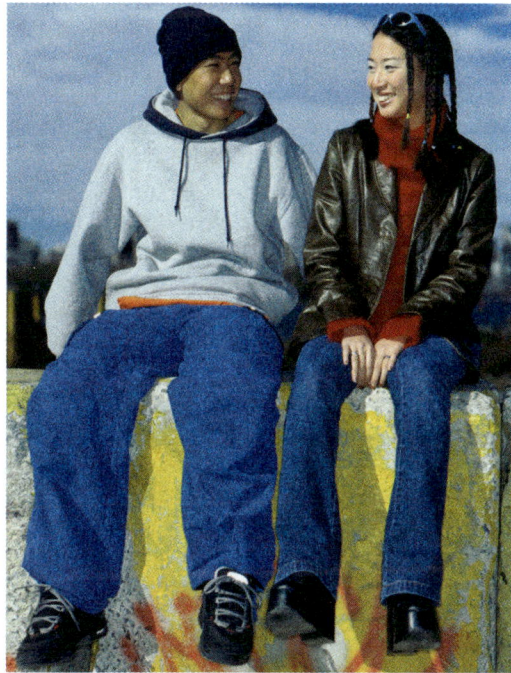

Use your clothing money to buy as many of the items on your list as you can. Start with the most important items. If you need a major clothing item, such as a winter coat, treat it as a one-time expense. Begin to budget for it several months in advance.

Check ads, catalogs, and several stores to estimate the prices of clothing items. Clothes often go on sale before and at the end of a season. You will find the lowest prices near the end of the season. However, buying this late in the season means you'll only have a limited wearing time before the seasons change. Choices may also be limited.

Use the following tips to help you stretch your clothing dollars and build your wardrobe:

- ☞ Check out resale clothing stores and thrift shops for used clothes at low prices. You can also buy lower-priced new clothes at clothing warehouses and discount centers. These options can save you quite a bit of money over shopping mall prices.
- ☞ Before you buy, try on garments in front of a full-length, three-way mirror. Check the fit and appearance. Move about and sit in the clothes to make sure they will be comfortable.
- ☞ Check the construction and quality of the clothes you buy. This matters most with used clothing or clothing at an off-price store. Some of these garments may be slightly flawed. Be sure any flaws won't affect fit or appearance.
- ☞ Read all labels and tags to learn what fabrics a garment contains and what care it needs. Avoid too many clothes that require dry cleaning. Dry-cleaning is costly. This can keep you from being able to use the clothes when you're short on money.
- ☞ For dress clothes, it is smart to choose one basic neutral color that will go with everything. Buy classic clothes that are right for various occasions and won't go out of style.
- ☞ Taking care of your clothes will help them last. Keep your clothes clean, pressed, and in good repair. Treat stains as they occur. Hang or fold clean clothes neatly and put them away.

Buying Furniture and Home Appliances

Suppose you rent a furnished apartment or live with your parents. You probably won't have to buy furniture or home appliances just yet. It's still good to learn how to shop for them. Sometime in the future you might make this type of purchase.

If you have an unfurnished apartment or house of your own, you may need to shop for these items. These major purchases can be more difficult than shopping for food or clothing. They involve more money. You want these items to last for many years, so you must choose carefully.

If you're buying furniture or an appliance, measure the space in your home to learn what will fit. Write the measurements on your shopping list. Take a tape measure with you to the store. This will help you avoid buying (and having to return) an item that is the wrong size.

Be sure to read all labels and owner's manuals from the manufacturer. These may describe how to use the item and what may happen if you misuse it. Many appliances also have special labels that state how much energy they will use. Add this cost to the final price when choosing which brand or model to buy. Ask what delivery and installation costs will apply. You'll need to add these expenses into your final cost, too.

When you own furniture or home appliances, your product may, at some time, need warranty service. To obtain this service, you will need proof of your purchase. You might need to show your sales receipt and warranty. Keep these important papers in your files. This way the information will be handy if you must call for warranty service.

Shopping at Sales

One way to save quite a bit of money is to shop at sales. Not every sale item is a bargain, though. With practice, you can learn to recognize real values. The guidelines on the next page can help.

☛ Take advantage of sale prices to save money on items you need and will use. If your budget allows, stock up on everyday items when sale prices are offered. This will cut your cost on items you had planned to buy anyway.

☛ Don't let price reductions tempt you to buy what you don't need or won't use. A $90 jacket that's on sale for $30 is not a bargain if it doesn't fit. Even at half price, a sewing machine isn't a bargain if you don't sew.

☛ Find out store policies on sale merchandise. Can you return or exchange sale items? If you return a sale item, will you receive a cash refund or only store credit? For cash refund, will you receive your full purchase price or only the current price of the item?

☛ Examine sale merchandise carefully. Be sure to get the right fit, color, and features. Items marked second, irregular, or as is, may be flawed. Check to be sure the defects will not interfere with your use of the product. This matters the most if you can't return sales items.

☛ Before you buy, calculate just what your savings will be. Saving 33 to 50 percent or more on something you need and want can be a real bargain. A smaller savings may or may not be a good deal, depending on the item. If sale items are soiled or damaged, add the cost of cleaning or repairs to the sale price.

☛ Plan your purchases to take advantage of seasonal sales. Most stores put certain kinds of items on sale at a set time each year. These sales are called seasonal sales. You may be able to save a lot of money if you can buy items you need at these sales. The exact schedule for seasonal sales will differ somewhat by area and store. Ads, salespeople, and store announcements can tell you what's on sale at a certain time of year.

Buying Services

Buying services differs from buying goods. With a service, you don't really know what you are getting until you receive it. For the most part, you buy on faith. This makes it important to know the reputation of any person or business that sells services you want to buy.

It takes special training, skills, or knowledge to provide some services. These include medical, dental, and vision care; car and home repairs; legal and financial advice; child care; and electronic and appliance servicing. You want qualified, trained people to provide these services. Look for a service provider with a solid reputation and the skills to do the job well. See Figure 4-15.

Find out about the person's qualifications. What education and training have they had? How much experience do they bring to the job? For important services, request the names of two or three customers you can call as references. Ask these customers if they've been pleased with the services they received. Choose service providers that others recommend.

4-15 When picking a doctor, shop around. Choose one who is well-qualified to meet your needs.

Suppose you need to purchase an expensive service, such as an auto repair. Ask for written estimates from at least three service providers. This has two benefits. First, it allows you to confirm the service is needed. Second, it lets you compare costs and service features among providers. Compare these estimates carefully and read all the details. Which provider offers the most reasonable price and makes you feel sure the job will be done well?

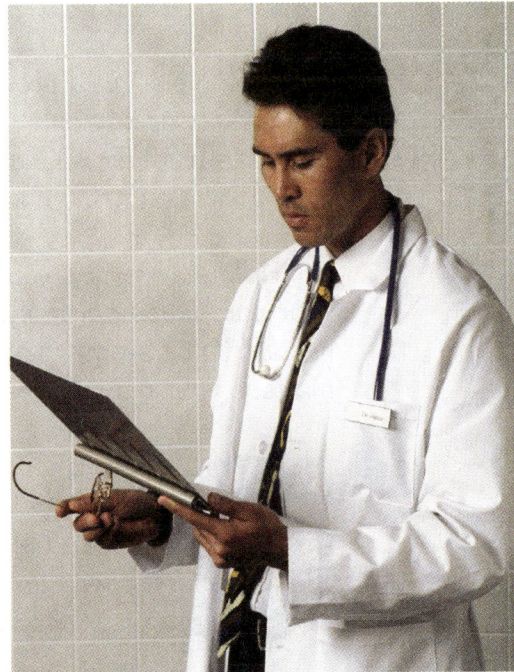

Some questions you can ask before you buy services include the following:

- Who would perform the service?
- How long will it take to complete?
- How much will it cost, and what does this price include?
- What happens if I'm not pleased with the outcome?

When you find a provider you can trust, return to this place in the future for any similar services you need. Building a relationship with this provider will help you avoid problems with the services you buy. It will also help you feel more comfortable.

No matter what you buy, it's good to take your time and plan your purchases carefully. With practice, you can develop the skills needed to be a smart shopper. Smart shopping will help you manage your money wisely. Both you and your family will benefit.

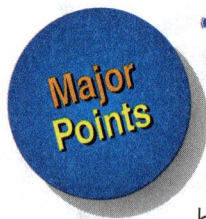

Major Points

- Shopping like a pro can help you stretch your dollars and get more of the goods and services you need and want. You can become a smart shopper who gets good values in the marketplace.
- Understanding the marketplace will help you become a better shopper. Many types of sellers are available. Some are better than others for certain situations. Learn the best places to buy the goods and services you need.
- It's important to evaluate the sellers you choose. Look for reliable sellers who will work hard to get and keep your business. When you find honest sellers, continue doing business with them.
- Finding reliable consumer information takes a little time and effort, but it is well worth it. Learn all you need to know about purchases before you buy. Read tags, labels, warranties, and manuals. Consult with salespeople and others you know. Look for information in ads, consumer articles, and government publications.
- Smart shopping takes several skills, which you can develop with practice. Some are general skills, while others apply more directly to buying goods or buying services. Mastering shopping skills will help you get the most from your money.

Chapter 5 Mastering Financial Tools

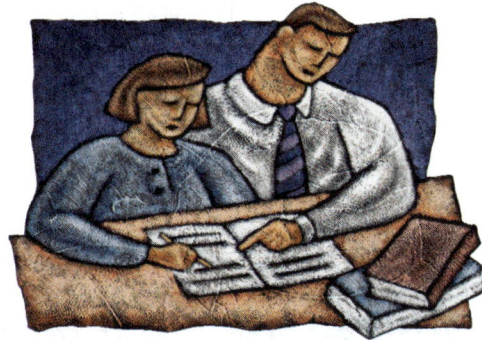

Budgeting and shopping skills aren't the only tools you will need for managing your money. Other financial tools can also help you manage money wisely. Three of these tools are credit, insurance, and personal bank accounts. These tools are powerful when used responsibly. They can help you reach financial goals and protect your money.

The first step is to learn what each tool is and how to use it. This chapter will teach you the basics of using credit, buying insurance, and managing a bank account. With practice, you can use these tools wisely to learn to support yourself financially.

Credit

Credit is an agreement that lets you buy now and pay later. The company that grants you the credit is the creditor. This company agrees to loan you money or let you make purchases as needed. You agree to repay this money in the future. Keep in mind that using credit means spending your future income. In time, you must pay for the goods and services you bought with credit.

You might wonder why creditors grant people credit. What's in it for them? The answer is interest, the fee you pay for the use of loaned money. Interest is the price you must pay for the privilege of using credit. When you think about using credit, add this cost into your purchase price.

The right to use credit is based on trust. To use credit, you must agree to pay what you owe plus the interest charged for the use of credit. The creditor trusts you to keep your word. Before you can get credit, you'll need to build a good credit rating. Your credit rating is an evaluation of your financial history. It shows whether you have a reputation of being willing and able to repay your debts. See Figure 5-1.

How to Get (and Keep) a Strong Credit Rating

To Establish a Strong Credit Rating

- Get and keep a job.
- Pay your bills promptly.
- Open a savings account and save regularly.
- Obtain credit at a local department store, make small purchases, and pay on time each month.
- Handle your financial matters in a businesslike way.

To Maintain a Strong Credit Rating

- Use only as much credit as you can comfortably repay.
- Meet all the terms of the credit contract or agreement.
- Pay your bills on time.
- Keep accurate records of charges, statements, and payments.
- Contact creditors if you cannot pay on time.
- Resolve billing errors promptly.

5-1 Your credit rating reflects your financial reputation. Work to build it and keep it strong.

When used wisely, credit can be a convenient and powerful tool. You can use it to help you manage your money. Be careful, though. Unwise use of credit can lead to serious problems. Your credit rating is your financial reputation. Learn more about what the credit process involves so you can protect your credit rating.

Before you use credit, make sure you understand what is expected of you. If you've already made some credit mistakes, you're not alone. Don't dwell on these mistakes. Instead, learn how to repair the damage and use money and credit more wisely in the future.

Sales Credit

Sales credit is one of the two basic types of credit. Sales credit lets you buy goods and services using a credit card or charge account.

You may be offered sales credit by a store that sells goods or services. An example would be a store charge account. You could use this type of credit to buy goods and services from the store issuing the account.

Credit cards are a second kind of sales credit. You might be issued a credit card by a bank or credit company. You could use this credit card to buy goods and services. Many credit cards can be used at a wide number of stores and service providers.

With sales credit, you might be offered one of three types of accounts. Creditors decide which type of account they will offer consumers.

A regular charge account lets you charge your purchases and be billed for them. You will receive a billing statement each month. This will show your charges, payments, and the total amount owed. You're expected to pay in full by the date shown on the statement (usually 25 days after the billing date). If you pay the full amount on time, no interest will be charged. Some credit card companies and stores offer regular charge accounts.

An installment account allows you to buy a costly item, such as furniture or a computer, over time. You pay the store a set amount each month until the purchase is paid in full. This type of account lets you use an item while paying for it. Legally, the creditor owns the item until you make all the payments. If you fail to pay, the creditor can repossess (take back) the item. If this happens, you will lose the item and all the money you had invested in it.

An installment account often requires a written contract. You may also have to make a down payment. This is an amount of cash you pay when you sign the contract. Until you have paid for the item, you will be charged interest.

The creditor must tell you how much you will be charged for the use of the credit. Finance charges include interest and any other amounts charged by the creditor as part of the credit agreement. Interest must be stated both as a dollar amount and as an annual percentage rate (APR). The APR is the actual rate of interest figured on a yearly basis. The APR for an installment account will vary. It may be as high as 18 to 24 percent. This amount will be added to the amount you owe. The interest and other finance charges will be included in your monthly payments.

The third type of account is a revolving credit account. This account lets you charge purchases to a stated dollar limit. The creditor sets this limit based on your credit rating. Most credit card companies, such as Visa, Mastercard, and Discover, offer revolving credit accounts. Some stores also issue this type of credit.

With this type of account, you are expected to pay a portion of the balance each month. This is called a minimum payment. This amount is set by the creditor based on how much you owe. It will appear on your statement. This is the amount you must pay, although you're welcome to pay more.

If you can pay more than the minimum payment, you will reduce your interest charges. If you can pay your account in full each month, you will pay no interest at all. If you pay less than the full amount, you'll pay finance charges on the unpaid balance. The interest charged is often 18 to 24 percent APR. This amount is added to your total.

Cash Credit

The second basic type of credit is cash credit. This is a loan in which you borrow money from a creditor. This loan might be made by a bank, savings and loan association, or credit union. Finance companies also make cash credit loans. You might borrow money to buy an expensive item, such as a car. If you're going to college, you might take student loans to pay for your classes. You would repay these loans over time.

A loan may be either unsecured or secured. An unsecured loan is made based on a person's credit rating alone. In this type of loan, you would sign a contract promising to repay. The terms of repayment would be stated in the contract. The creditor trusts you to keep your word. Only people with strong credit ratings can get unsecured loans.

A secured loan is one in which you must offer some sort of security for the creditor. This may be collateral, a cosigner, or both. Collateral is an item of value you own and pledge to the creditor to secure the loan. For example, if you borrow to buy a car, the car would be security for the loan. If you fail to repay the loan, the creditor could repossess the car. A cosigner is a person with a strong credit rating who signs a loan contract with you. This person promises to pay the debt if you fail to do so. Your cosigner puts his or her credit rating on the line to guarantee the loan will be paid.

By faithfully repaying a loan as agreed, you strengthen your credit history. Each time you pay off a loan as agreed, your credit rating improves. You prove you can keep your word. In the future, it will be easier for you to get the credit you need.

Loans vary by the way you repay them. Three types of loans are the installment loan, the single payment loan, and a credit card or check credit loan. The installment loan calls for regular monthly payments. Car loans and student loans are examples. The loan will include finance charges. These charges will depend on the amount you borrow, the interest rate, and the length of time you take to repay. See Figure 5-2.

With a single payment loan, you repay the entire loan in one payment at a set time in the future. An example is a small cash loan you take out from the bank. Finance charges will apply to this

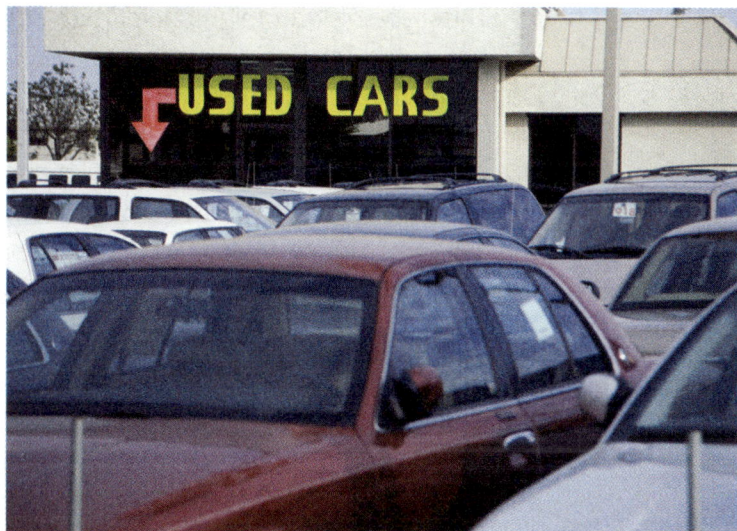

5-2 Buying a car is a wise use of credit if you can afford the car and can repay the installment loan as agreed.

type of loan. Some creditors subtract these charges from the money you borrow before giving it to you. Others add the finance charges to the amount you must repay. The amount of the finance charges depends on how much you borrow and the interest rate.

A credit card or check credit loan is a little different. You use your credit card or a check to borrow money from the creditor. The creditor sets the terms for this kind of loan and enters an agreement with you. This agreement states how much you can borrow and how you will repay it. If you use a credit card to borrow money, this is called a cash advance. In some cases, the bank will accept a special check you've written for this type of loan. The terms of this type of loan are very much like those of a revolving charge account. Finance charges apply to the unpaid balance each month.

One type of check credit loan to avoid is the payday loan. It may also be called a cash advance loan, check advance loan, or delayed deposit loan. Many companies will loan you money against your future paychecks. The cost for this service is quite high, however.

In this type of loan, you write a post-dated check (check with a future date on it). The lender agrees to wait until that date to deposit your check. At the time you write the check, the lender gives you the money minus a substantial fee.

This type of loan might help in an emergency, but shouldn't be used on a regular basis. Very often, consumers who take this kind of loan think it will help them in a pinch. When they take this loan, they are receiving (and often spending) their future income. This puts them in a bind. It may tempt them to take another payday loan to get through the next pay period. Soon, taking these loans is a habit and the consumer loses a large amount of money paying for this service. This money could be better spent meeting other financial needs.

Credit Costs

When making credit decisions, keep in mind that credit comes at a price. For the item you want to purchase, is the cost of credit worth it to you? To answer this question, you must know how much you will pay for credit each time you use it. The following three factors will influence your credit cost:

- ☞ how much credit you use
- ☞ what interest rate (APR) rate is charged
- ☞ how much time you take to repay

Credit costs increase with the amount of credit used. You'll pay more interest (given as an APR) for a large loan than for a small loan. This is because the APR is a percentage of the total amount of credit you use. Suppose you took a loan and repaid it in 12 monthly payments at 18 percent APR. If the loan was $500, the interest would be $50.08. For a $1,000 loan, the interest would climb to $110.01.

Credit costs rise as the APR increases. You will pay more for credit with a high APR than for credit with a lower APR. A higher APR means you will pay a higher percentage of the total credit used. Suppose you borrow $500 and repay it in 12 monthly payments. At 18 percent APR, the interest would be $50.08. If the rate rose to 24 percent, the interest would be $67.36.

Credit costs increase over time. A creditor will charge interest until you've repaid your debt in full. Keep your repayment time as short as possible. This will reduce the amount of interest paid. Suppose you borrow $500 at 18 percent APR. If you repay it in 24 monthly payments, the interest would be $99.44. For 36 monthly payments, the interest would rise to $150.88.

Keep these three principles in mind when you use credit. Under the law, creditors must tell you the cost of credit. They must state it both as a dollar amount and as an APR. This makes it easy to compare costs and interest rates from one creditor to the next. Shop for the lowest rates among creditors before accepting credit.

Credit Contracts

By signing a credit contract, you are saying you accept its terms. (A credit contract is sometimes called an agreement). After you sign, these terms are legally binding. Under the law, you must now follow the contract. This is why you need to understand what you are agreeing to do before you sign.

When you apply for credit, you should receive a credit contract. This paper should explain the terms of the credit offer. It should describe your responsibilities and those of the creditor. Read the contract carefully. Underline any terms or phrases you don't understand. Find out what these terms mean so you can decide whether to agree to them. If you need help understanding the terms of the contract, seek advice from someone with experience in financial matters.

The contract should state the APR and dollar cost of the credit. It will also outline the terms of repayment. These include the amounts due, payment due dates, and penalties for late or missed payments. Study the contract to learn what will happen if you pay late or miss a payment. Examine the sample contract in Figure 5-3.

KEEP THIS NOTICE FOR FUTURE USE
BELK RETAIL CHARGE AGREEMENT

1. Each time I receive the monthly statement (at about the same time each month) I will decide whether to pay the New Balance of the account in full or in part. If full payment of the New Balance shown on the statement is received, by BELK, by the Payment Due Date, No FINANCE CHARGE will be added to the account. Any month I choose not to pay the New Balance in full, I will make at least the minimum partial payment listed on the statement as Minimum Payment Now Due. Each month the Minimum Payment Due will be calculated according to the following schedule:

If New Balance Is	Less Than $10	$10-100	$101-150	$151-200	$201-250	$251-300	Over $300
Minimum Monthly Payment Is	Balance	$10	$15	$20	$25	$30	⅒ of account balance rounded to next highest $5 increment

2. If payment in full is not received by the Payment Due Date, I agree to pay a FINANCE CHARGE at the rate described below for my State of residence.

Annual Percentage Rate for Purchases	10% to 21% (see table below)		
State of Residence	Periodic Rate	Annual Percentage Rate	Portion of Average Daily Balance To Which Applied
DE., KY., VA., MS., GA., OK., MD.	1.75%	21%	ENTIRE
NC., PA., TN., FL., TX and all other states	1.50%	18%	ENTIRE
AL.	1.75%	21%	$750 or less
	1.5%	18%	over $750
WV.	1.5%	18%	$750 or less
	1.0%	12%	over $750
SC.	1.75%	21%	$650 or less
	1.5%	18%	over $650
MO.	1.5%	18%	$1,000 or less
	1.0%	12%	over $1,000
AR.	.083%	10%	ENTIRE
Grace Period:	You have until the next billing date which on average is 23 days if the balance is paid in full, before a finance charge will be imposed.		
Method of Computing the Average Daily Balance.	Average Daily Balance Method: We figure a portion of the finance charge on your account by applying the periodic rate to the "average daily balance" of your account (including current transactions). To get the "average daily balance", we take the beginning balance of your account each day, add any new purchases and subtract any payments or credits, and unpaid finance charges. This gives us the daily balance. Then, we add up all the daily balances for the billing cycle and divide the total by the number of days in the billing cycle. This gives us the "average daily balance".		

3. Credit for returned merchandise will not substitute for a payment.

4. BELK has the right to amend the terms and conditions of this agreement by advising me of its intentions to do so in a manner and to the extent required by law.

5. If any payment is not received by BELK by the Payment Due Date, the full unpaid balance of the account may, at the option of Belk, become due and payable. If the account is referred for collection by Belk to any outside agency and/or attorney, who is not a salaried employee of BELK, I will, to the extent permitted by law, pay all costs including attorney fees.

6. BELK reserves the right to charge a handling fee, not to exceed the amount permitted by law, on any check used for payment on the account that is returned by the bank for insufficient funds or otherwise unpaid.

7. If this is a joint account, both of us agree to be bound by the terms of this agreement and each of us agrees to be jointly and severally liable for payment of all purchases made under this agreement.

8. The credit card issued to me in connection with this account remains the property of BELK and I will surrender it upon request. I understand that BELK is not obligated to extend to me any credit and, without prior notice, may refuse to allow me to make any purchase or incur any other charge on my account. Such refusal will not affect my obligation to pay the balance existing on my account at the time.

9. If any provision of this agreement is found to be invalid or unenforceable, the remainder of this agreement shall not be affected thereby, and the rest of this agreement shall be valid and enforced to the fullest extent permitted by law. No delay, omission, or waiver in the enforcement of any provision of this agreement by BELK will be deemed to be a waiver of any subsequent breach of such provision or of any other provision of this agreement.

10. I hereby authorize BELK, or any credit bureau employed by BELK, to investigate references, statements, and other data contained on my application or obtained from me or any other source pertaining to my credit worthiness. I will furnish further information if requested. I authorize BELK to furnish information concerning its credit experience with me to credit reporting agencies and others who may lawfully receive such information.

11. Except as provided in paragraph 2 above, this agreement will be governed by the laws of the State of North Carolina.

5-3 A credit contract can seem like a lot of "fine print," but it's important to read and understand every word before you sign.

Before you sign the contract, take a last careful look. Be sure you understand all you are agreeing to do. Be sure all the blanks are filled in or crossed out so nothing can be added or changed later. Sign only if you are sure you can carry out the terms of the contract.

Laws That Protect You

When you use credit, you have many legal rights. See Figure 5-4 for a list of important consumer protection laws. These laws will protect you as you use credit.

First, the law requires creditors to tell you certain facts before you sign a credit contract. This includes information about finance charges, payments, penalties, and other contract terms. With this information, you can make wise credit choices.

Creditors must not discriminate when giving credit. They must offer or deny you credit based only on your credit rating. You can't be turned down because of your gender, marital status, ethnic group, religion, or age. Whether you've ever been on public aid can't be a factor, either.

The law states that credit reports must be accurate. It's illegal for an agency to report false information about you. Suppose you're denied credit because of a credit report. You have the right to receive the name and address of the agency that made the report. Request a copy of this report and check it for mistakes. If you find false information, contact the reporting agency. The agency must then correct the report. A new report must be sent to anyone who received the first one.

Laws also protect you from unfair credit billing practices. If you disagree with your bill, you have the right to take this up with the creditor. Until the matter is settled, the creditor can't collect the amount in dispute. This holds true even if your debt is sold to another creditor.

Finally, creditors cannot use unfair methods to collect debt. It's good to know and stand up for your legal rights concerning the use of credit. This helps you protect yourself as a consumer.

Consumer Credit Laws

Law	Protection It Provides
Truth in Lending Law	Requires creditors to tell you certain details about using credit including ✤ amount financed or borrowed ✤ total number, amount, and due dates of payments ✤ finance charges in dollar amount and annual percentage rate (APR) ✤ all charges not included in the finance charge ✤ penalties for late payment, default, or prepayment
Equal Credit Opportunity Act	Prohibits creditors from discriminating against you based on your gender, marital status, race, national origin, religion, age, or receipt of public aid
Fair Credit Reporting Act	Requires information on credit reports to be accurate and private Gives you the right to know the name of any credit agency that has given false information about you and to have that information corrected
Fair Credit Billing Act	Protects you against unfair billing practices Tells you how to resolve billing errors and disputes Prohibits creditors from trying to collect amounts in dispute
Fair Debt Collection Practices Act	Prohibits creditors from ✤ revealing or publicizing your debt to others ✤ contacting you at inconvenient times or places ✤ making repeated or anonymous phone calls ✤ using threats or abusive language ✤ making false or misleading statements about their identity or the consequences of failing to pay ✤ collecting unauthorized fees or charging you for calls and telegrams

5-4 Consumer credit laws protect you when you use credit. Being familiar with these laws helps you protect your rights.

Managing Credit

Credit is a resource you need to manage wisely. When you use credit, you are spending your future income. Managing credit takes self-control, which includes the following:

- planning credit purchases before you buy
- using credit responsibly to build and maintain a strong credit rating
- keeping your word about repaying your credit debt on time
- maintaining detailed records of your credit use and payments you make
- paying close attention to billing errors and reporting them promptly
- avoiding serious credit mistakes
- never giving your card number over the phone unless you made the call
- shredding bank and credit statements and credit card offers before throwing them away

Deciding When to Use Credit

Think about whether using credit for this purpose is a good idea for you. Weigh the pros and cons of using it. Consider your other options. See Figure 5-5.

Weighing the Use of Credit

Advantages	Disadvantages	Alternatives to Credit
❖ Credit allows you to use goods and services as you pay for them.	❖ Using credit reduces future income.	❖ If you already have savings, use some of your savings to buy the item.
❖ Using credit helps you buy costly items that you could not pay for all at once.	❖ When you use credit, you will likely face finance charges. Over time, these can be costly.	❖ Save now and buy later if you can often do without or postpone the purchase.
❖ Credit is a source of cash for emergencies and unexpected expenses.	❖ When you have credit, you may be tempted to spend more than you can afford.	❖ Buy on a layaway plan.
❖ Credit is a convenient way to pay for certain goods and services.	❖ Misusing credit can cause serious financial problems.	❖ Find a less costly substitute item (such as used rather than new) you can afford.

5-5 Good money managers take the time to decide whether using credit for a particular purchase is wise. Keep these points in mind as you make credit choices.

If you choose to use credit, it's smart to set some rules about how you will use it. First, decide for what reasons you will use it. Wise ways you could use credit include the following:

- ☞ meeting emergency expenses
- ☞ reaching a long-term financial goal, such as an education
- ☞ taking advantage of sale prices without breaking your budget
- ☞ buying an expensive item you need right away, such as an appliance or a car

You might choose to use credit for one, some, or all of these reasons. Whatever rule you make, try to stick to it. This will ensure you make the best use possible of your credit dollars.

When Not to Use Credit

Risky uses of credit can lead to financial problems. It isn't wise to borrow or spend more than you can afford to repay. Be honest with yourself about how much of your budget you can devote to credit payments each month.

Don't use credit to live beyond your means. Going on a shopping spree can be fun at the time, but it can take months, or even years, to recover financially. Avoid the temptation to buy just because you can. This is especially true of items you don't really need. In time, you must pay for all these items. Where will the money come from to pay your credit bill? Avoid using credit unless you can answer this question.

Understanding Your Statement

If you use credit cards or store charge accounts, you will receive a monthly billing statement. You may get one for a loan, too. Take some time to learn what information these statements contain. See the sample statement in Figure 5-6.

Save the sales slips and receipts for all your credit card or store charge account purchases. Keep these on file along with your monthly statements. Check each statement against your records. Contact the creditor right away if you notice an error or a difference. Also, let the creditor know if you have questions about your account.

The total amount you can charge to your account.

The amount of credit that is currently available in your account.

CHARGE CARD STATEMENT

$ WRITE IN THE AMOUNT OF YOUR PAYMENT

IMPORTANT!   1. Return the portion of your statement with your check; please do not fold or bend.   2. Write your account number on the face of your check.   3. Make checks payable to Charge Card.

ACCOUNT NUMBER	BILLING DATE	PAYMENT DUE DATE	NEW BALANCE	MINIMUM PAYMENT DUE
5211-7627-58	11-28-xx	12-23-x x	457.80	23.00
4211-576-275-8				

PLEASE BE SURE OUR MAILING ADDRESS ON THE REVERSE SIDE APPEARS IN THE WINDOW OF THE RETURN ENVELOPE.

Account number or numbers.

130   MARY PHELPS
123. W. TAFT DR.
SOUTH HOLLAND, IL 60473

IMPORTANT- PLEASE WRITE YOUR
ACCOUNT NUMBER ON YOUR CHECK.
730008447
5211762754RL 0045780000500000002300

FOR CHANGE OF ADDRESS PLEASE PRINT | NEW STREET ADDRESS | PHONE NO.
CITY | STATE | ZIP CODE

RETAIN THIS PORTION FOR YOUR RECORDS

The portion of the statement to be returned with your payment.

The date each transaction was made.

Account Number	Credit Limit	Available Credit	Past Due Amount	BILLING DATE
5211-7627-58 4211-576-275-8	2,000.00	1,542.20		11-28-xx

The date the statement was prepared.

TRAN. DATE	POSTING DATE	REFERENCE NUMBER	TRANSACTION DESCRIPTION	TRANSACTION AMOUNT
1021	1104	V00917073	THOM BEESON LT DEERFIELD IL	11.84
1021	1111	V01629355	REOS GARDEN CENTER INC NORTHBROOK IL	27.72
1024	1101	MH0634591	WILMETTE BOOTERY INC WILMETTE IL	30.74
1028	1107	MH1226125	THE PUMP ROOM CHICAGO IL	26.50
1101	1108	MH1320621	OZARK AIRLINES WATERLOO IL	94.00
1103	1107	V01218714	CRATE&BARREL NORTH INC WILMETTE IL	15.69
1105	1113	MH1854.15	CLOTHES CORNER WILMETTE IL	42.40
1107	1115	MH2065221	INITIAL IT WINNETKA IL	12.72
1108	1114	MH1939852	HERMANS SPTNG GDS 16 HIGHPARK IL	54.50
1108	1113	M3182749.19	DOMINICKS #62 NORTHFIELD IL	107.11
1121	1121	D990004.3	PAYMENT THANK YOU	264.13CR

The date each transaction was posted.

A number that describes each transaction that was made.

Amount of each item charged to your account.

The place each transaction took place.

PERIODIC RATE: PURCHASES AND CASH ADVANCES 1.5%.
ANNUAL PERCENTAGE RATE   PURCHASES AND CASH ADVANCES 18%.

The minimum payment that must be paid.

The annual percentage rate charged on your account.

PREVIOUS BALANCE	AVERAGE DAILY BALANCE	FINANCE CHARGE	NEW BALANCE	Minimum Payment
286.63	471.90	7.08	457.80	23.00

YOU MAY AT ANY TIME PAY ALL OR PART OF THE TOTAL BALANCE OWING ON YOUR ACCOUNT.

For Customer Service Ca	Charge Transactions	PAYMENTS	CREDITS	PAYMENT DUE DATE
312-555-4110	428.22	264.13	.00	12-23-xx

The date by which you must pay at least the minimum payment.

Additional FINANCE CHARGE on purchases may be avoided if total NEW BALANCE is paid in full by PAYMENT DUE DATE.
You are not required to pay any amount which you properly notify us as in dispute pending our compliance with applicable law.
NOTICE: SEE REVERSE SIDE FOR IMPORTANT INFORMATION

The balance remaining at the beginning of the current billing period.

Balance remaining at the end of the current billing period.

Total amount of charges made during the billing period.

Total amount of payments made during the billing period.

Total amount of credits added to your account during the billing period.

The total of each day's outstanding balance in the monthly billing period divided by the number of days in the monthly billing period.

The amount of finance charges added to your account.

5-6 This is a typical credit account statement. Yours may differ slightly, but should contain most of the same information.

Dealing with Credit Problems

Unwise use of credit can quickly lead to serious problems. These problems can have serious and lasting results. Learn to recognize credit problems early and solve them right away. Waiting can make things even worse.

Follow the repayment terms of your credit agreement. Paying the full amount on time can build your credit rating. Avoid paying late, missing a payment, or sending less than the amount due. This can damage your credit rating. It also greatly raises the cost of credit. You may be charged late fees or your APR may be increased. Late fees or interest that put your account over the limit will create even more fees. Read your credit agreement to learn the exact consequences for late and missed payments.

There may be a time when you just can't pay the full amount by the due date. If this happens, call your creditor right away. Don't wait until the payment is overdue. Give the creditor as much notice as you can. Try to make an arrangement with the creditor to pay what you can. Ask if you can do this without penalties or fees. (You may avoid them by calling well in advance.) This responsible approach can help protect your credit rating.

If you're having a hard time paying your bills, take a close look at your finances. What role does your use of credit play? Ask yourself the questions in Figure 5-7. Answering yes to these questions indicates you may have a problem.

Act fast to get your finances under control. This will help you avoid further problems. Credit counseling may help. Try the Consumer Credit Counseling Service nearest you. This nonprofit agency is run by the National Foundation for Consumer Credit, which has offices throughout the country. Visit nfcc.org or check your local phone book to find an office near you. Ask to talk to a qualified counselor who can advise you about your finances. This person can talk to your creditors and help you set a plan to repay your debts. He or she can also help you make a plan to avoid future debt problems. This counseling costs little or nothing.

Credit Danger Checklist

Complete this checklist about your use of credit. If you answer YES to a few of these questions, think about how you could improve your use of credit. If you answer YES to many or all of these questions, seek help at once.

YES	NO	
❑	❑	Have you experienced a reduction or loss of income recently?
❑	❑	Do you often use money intended for one purpose for another?
❑	❑	Do you often spend impulsively and later regret your purchases?
❑	❑	Do you use credit or dip into savings for unessential items?
❑	❑	Do you tend to overestimate income and underestimate expenses?
❑	❑	Do you find it difficult to meet routine expenses?
❑	❑	Do you use credit to meet routine monthly expenses?
❑	❑	Do you often receive overdue notices on bills?
❑	❑	Do you have trouble paying your bills on time?
❑	❑	Do you pay only the minimum payment each month?
❑	❑	Do you borrow from one creditor to pay another?
❑	❑	Do you charge more on your credit accounts each month than you pay?
❑	❑	Do you figure the future can take care of itself rather than making a plan?
❑	❑	Do you feel your financial situation is beyond your control?

5-7 Are you on the brink of credit disaster? Take this quiz to find out.

Seek advice only from a reputable counseling service. Avoid businesses that offer debt consolidation (pooling). These companies want to loan you money to pool your bills. The interest on these loans is very high. These businesses are out to make money. You cannot rely upon them to do what's best for you. Debt consolidation might do you more harm than good.

Insurance

What would happen to your finances in a crisis? Could you afford the costs of an accident that caused severe injury, disability, or death? Could you repair or replace property that was damaged or stolen? How would you pay for medical care to treat a major illness? Each of these events can cause a great deal of financial loss. See Figure 5-8. This loss can devastate a family who is not prepared for it.

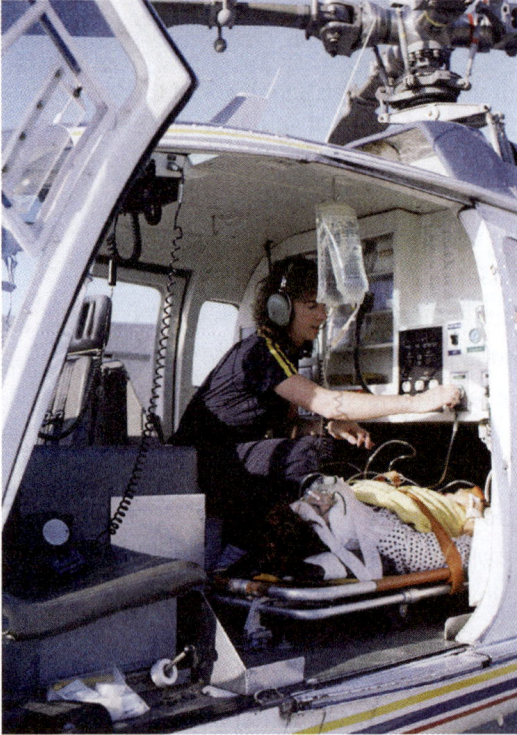

5-8 For a family without insurance, a medical emergency can lead to financial hardship.

To protect yourself from such losses, you might want to buy insurance. This is an agreement between you and an insurance company to share the risks of a financial loss. The fee you must pay for insurance is called a premium. For this cost, the insurance company agrees to pay some of the costs if such a loss occurs.

When you buy insurance, you receive an insurance policy. This is your contract with the insurance company. It proves you are protected by the company. It also states the terms of your coverage, or protection. Each policy lists certain losses as covered losses. The insurance company will pay you for these types of loss. Policies also list exclusions. These are losses the policy does not cover.

Your policy will also state the deductible amount. This is the part of your losses you must pay before you can collect from the insurance company. For example, if your deductible is $500, you must pay the first $500 of a covered loss. After you pay this amount, the insurance company must pay for the rest of the loss up to the limits stated in the policy. Usually, you can choose the deductible amount. A policy with a high deductible will have a lower premium than one with a lower deductible.

You may wonder why an insurance company would agree to pay your losses. The company sells policies to thousands of people. All these people pay premiums. Very few actually suffer losses. When there are no losses, the company keeps all the premiums. When losses do occur, the company has more than enough money to pay losses and still show a profit.

As a teen parent, it will likely take you some time and hard work to obtain costly items. Check into insuring these items. This will protect you against financial loss. Otherwise, a crisis could wipe away your possessions. Replacing them would be costly, if not impossible. Insurance can give you peace of mind. Basic types of insurance include the following:

☛ Automobile insurance protects you from the financial risks of owning a car. In all 50 states, the law requires car owners to have auto insurance. If you own a car, you must carry at least two types of coverage. These are called bodily injury liability and property damage liability. These pay for the losses of others caused by your car. Covered losses might include the injury of others or damage to their property.

You must carry the types and amounts of auto insurance the law requires. Keep proof of your insurance in the car at all times. If you can't prove you have insurance, you can be fined and ordered to appear in court. Your driver's license or car registration could be suspended.

If you're repaying a car loan, the creditor may require you to carry more insurance than the law does. Check your credit contract to see what insurance you must have. You can also choose to buy added insurance coverage. This will protect you, your passengers, and your car even further. See Figure 5-9.

☛ Homeowner's insurance protects your home and possessions against the risks listed in the policy. When you buy a home, most mortgage lenders will require you to carry some type of homeowner's insurance. If you don't own your home, you may choose renter's insurance. This type of insurance protects your belongings.

☛ Life insurance protects your family against the loss of income that would occur if you died. You pay a premium for this protection. In the policy, you would name the person or people you want to receive the money. These people are called your beneficiaries. Often, parents name their children as beneficiaries. In this way, parents provide some money for their children to have after they die.

Types of Auto Insurance Coverage

Required by Law	❖ **Bodily injury liability** pays the damages when you're responsible for an accident in which others are injured or killed.
	❖ **Property damage liability** pays the damages when you're responsible for an auto accident in which the property of others is damaged.
Often Required for Car Loan	❖ **Collision insurance** pays for damage to your car resulting from an auto accident.
	❖ **Comprehensive physical damage insurance** pays for loss or damage to your car that is not caused by an auto accident. It includes theft, vandalism, fire, and other listed hazards.
Additional Options	❖ **Uninsured motorist insurance** pays for injuries caused by an uninsured or hit-and-run driver.
	❖ **Medical payments coverage** pays for insured persons' medical expenses that are caused by a car accident.

5-9 When you buy a car, you must carry the insurance required by law and by the lender that you're repaying. You can buy additional coverage if you need it.

There are different types of life insurance. Term insurance pays if you die while the policy is in force. It builds no cash value, but it provides the most coverage for the least amount of money. A cash value policy is one that pays at death but also builds cash value over the life of the policy.

☞ Health insurance helps you pay for the medical care you need to be healthy. It may cover preventative care. This is care that prevents problems or catches them early. A share of the costs for the care you need from a doctor or hospital would also be covered. Some policies cover prescription drugs, too. Health insurance matters most when you have a major illness or injury. The costs for being in the hospital or having surgery are very high.

Most adults get health insurance through their employers. Some companies pay all or part of the premiums for their employees. Employers may offer group health insurance, which is the most affordable. Two common kinds are health maintenance organizations (HMOs) and preferred provider organizations (PPOs). These benefits may be offered only to full-time workers. Until you work full-time, employer-sponsored insurance may not be an option for you.

If you can't get insurance through an employer, you may want to look into other options. Find out if your baby's father can include you or the baby on his coverage. Ask your parents whether you are covered under their insurance.

If your income is low, find out whether you qualify for Medicaid. If so, you and your child could get the health care you need at little or no cost. You can apply for Medicaid at your local social services office.

Buying more insurance than you really need can be a waste of money. Talk with more than one insurance agent before buying. Be sure to find out exactly how much coverage you need. The more you have to lose, the more insurance you'll need. Use insurance wisely to protect yourself and your family from financial loss. This could be your key for saving your family from financial ruin during a crisis.

Personal Bank Accounts

As a teen parent, you know the value of money management. A personal savings or checking account with a bank is a tool you can use to keep your money safe. Through your account, you can also keep track of the money you spend and receive each month. Building a relationship with your bank can also be helpful.

A bank's primary functions are to receive, transfer, and lend money. The bank serves consumers, businesses, and the government. Depending on where you live, there may be many banks, a few banks, or only one bank. The number of options may limit your choice. If your area has more than one bank, compare the services and accounts offered by each before deciding. Meet with a personal banker at each bank. Ask questions about what the bank offers.

Even within the same bank, there may be several types of savings and checking accounts. Have the banker explain each type. Be sure to ask for more details if you don't understand. Also ask for brochures with basic information about the accounts. You can take these brochures home and compare banks or accounts. Choosing a bank and a type of account is a big decision. Take your time to choose what will work best for you.

Savings Accounts

A savings account is a bank account where you can keep your money safe for future use. If you can save even a little money, think about opening a savings account. It would be much safer than keeping the money with you or storing it in your house. You might lose the money or someone might steal it. You'd also be more easily tempted to spend the money instead of saving it. Having a savings account reduces these risks.

When shopping for a savings account, there is much you will want to know. Ask what amount is required to open the account. If you don't have this much at first, be patient. Keep saving until you have enough to open an account. Ask if there is a minimum balance that must remain in the account at all times. If so, what fees or penalties apply for failing to keep this much in the account? What rules apply when you deposit (put money in the account) or withdraw (take money from the account) your money? Learning how different savings accounts work will help you choose the one that's right for you.

With many savings accounts, you will earn money by having money on deposit. This is called interest income. Some savings accounts don't pay interest income. An account that does may require a larger minimum balance to open the account. If so, start by opening a savings account that doesn't pay interest. Once you've saved enough, you can move this money to an interest-bearing account. See Figure 5-10 for more guidelines about the interest income paid on savings.

If you keep depositing money into your account, in time you will build quite a savings. This will help you meet unexpected expenses that arise. It will also help you meet long-term financial goals.

Making the Most of Interest Income

When shopping for a savings account, keep in mind the following guidelines about interest income:

❖ Most savings accounts pay *compound interest*. This means you earn interest income both on the money you have in the account and any interest income you've already earned. This type of account pays more than one that pays *simple interest*, where the interest income is always figured only on the money you have in the account.

❖ Your bank chooses how often to compound interest income. It can do this continuously, daily, monthly, or annually. You will earn more interest income as the frequency of compounding increases.

❖ You will earn more interest income as the interest rate paid by the bank increases. As the interest rate rises, you will earn a higher percentage of interest income on your savings.

❖ You will earn more interest income if you keep your money in savings longer. If you take money out of the account, the balance on which you will earn interest income is lower.

5-10 Earning interest income is the biggest benefit of most savings accounts. These guidelines tell you how to earn the highest amount of interest income possible.

Checking Accounts

A checking account is an account that lets you deposit money and then write checks on the account. This provides a safe place to keep your money. It can also be a very convenient way to pay for goods, services, and bills. A checking account can also provide a record of spending. Your cancelled checks can serve as proof of payment.

Most banks offer several types of checking accounts. These accounts will differ in the following ways:

☛ how much you must deposit to open the account

☛ how much money you must keep in the account at all times

☛ how many checks you can write

☛ what fee (if any) is charged per check

☛ what the fees and penalties are if you fall below this balance

☛ what other fees might apply to the account

☛ whether the account earns interest income

Ask a personal banker to explain each checking account offered. This person can also advise you which type of account would best meet your needs.

With your checking account, you may receive a card to help you manage your money. It might be an ATM card or a debit card. With these cards, you will have more options about how you deposit and withdraw money from your account. These cards also present some risks, though.

Once you've chosen which type of account you want, you'll be asked to sign a signature card. Sign the card the way you intend to sign your name for all your financial transactions. This will be the only signature the bank will honor on your checks and withdrawal slips.

After you open an account, you'll need to order checks printed with your name, address, and account number. Order your first box of checks through the bank. For later boxes, you might be able to use other check printing services. Many of these services offer checks at a lower cost. Ask your bank if this is an option.

Included with your checks will be a checkbook register. This is a small booklet in which you can keep track of your checks, deposits, and the balance in your account. See Figure 5-11. It is important to write everything that happens with your account in this register. This helps you keep track of your money and avoid overdrawing the account. You overdraw the account if you write a check for more money than you have in your account.

Overdrawing the account can have serious consequences. First, you are charged a fee by the bank each time this occurs. Next, the bank might refuse to pay your check. If they don't pay the check, you may face a charge from the company to which you wrote the check. These charges can add up quickly and greatly reduce the amount of money in your account. If you're not aware of the problem immediately, you might write more checks that "bounce." This can be

RECORD ALL CHARGES OR CREDITS THAT AFFECT YOUR ACCOUNT

NUMBER	DATE	CODE	DESCRIPTION OF TRANSACTION	PAYMENT/DEBIT (−)	√ T	FEE (IF ANY) (−)	PAYMENT/CREDIT (+)	BALANCE
	3/1		Opening Balance				100 00	100 00
								100 00
101	3/2		Lee's Grocery	15 32				15 32
			Groceries					84 68
	3/3	ATM	Cash Withdrawal	20 00				20 00
								64 68
102	3/4		The Baby Place	11 75				11 75
			Baby Supplies					52 93
	3/6	DC	No Limits	35 13				35 13
			Jeans					17 80
	3/8	D	Deposit				130 00	130 00
								147 80
103	3/9		Lee's Grocery	18 35				18 35
			Groceries					129 45
	3/11	AP	Unified Utilities	23 07				23 07
			Electric Bill					106 38
	3/14	DC	Mary's Dept. Store	34 60				34 60
			Baby Carrier					71 78
104	3/16		Richard's CDs	21 20				21 20
			CD					50 58
	3/22	D	Deposit				130 00	130 00
								180 58
105	3/26		Lee's Grocery	47 58				47 58
			Groceries					133 00
	3/29	ATM	Cash Withdrawal	30 00				30 00
								103 00
106	3/30		Dr. Harvey	65 00				65 00
			Dental Checkup					38 00
	4/1	D	Deposit				130 00	130 00
								168 00
	4/3		Service Charge	5 00				5 00
								163 00

*USE THESE CODES WHEN RECORDING YOUR NON-CHECK TRANSACTIONS

D = DEPOSIT   DC = DEBIT CARD   ATM = TELLER MACHINE   AP = AUTOMATIC PAYMENT   TT = TELEPHONE TRANSFER   T = TAX DEDUCTIBLE   O = OTHER

5-11 Keep a detailed record in your checkbook register. This way you will know how much money you have in your account at all times.

a costly mistake—one that can take a lot of time and money to fix. Take the time to keep good records so this won't happen to you.

In addition to keeping records, you'll need to learn certain tasks to manage your checking account. These are not difficult tasks, but it may take you a little time to learn them. Soon you'll be skilled at endorsing checks, making deposits, writing checks, and balancing your checkbook. These skills will help you transfer money into and out of your account with ease.

Endorsing a Check

When you receive a check, you will want to cash it or deposit it into your account. To do this, you'll need to endorse the check, or sign your name on the back of it. Some banks also ask you to write your account number as part of the endorsement. Always use pen to sign a check. This way, no one can tamper with your endorsement. Use the same signature you gave on your signature card. Finally, choose the best type of endorsement for this check. See Figure 5-12.

A blank endorsement includes only your signature (and perhaps your account number). Anyone can cash a check that is endorsed in this way. Use this endorsement only at the time and place you want to cash or deposit the check. This reduces the risk of others cashing your check if it is lost or stolen.

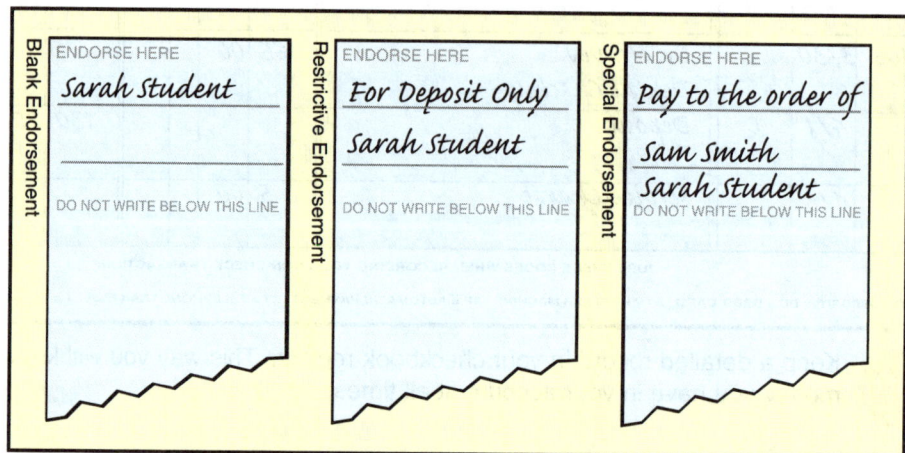

Blank Endorsement	Restrictive Endorsement	Special Endorsement
ENDORSE HERE Sarah Student DO NOT WRITE BELOW THIS LINE	ENDORSE HERE For Deposit Only Sarah Student DO NOT WRITE BELOW THIS LINE	ENDORSE HERE Pay to the order of Sam Smith Sarah Student DO NOT WRITE BELOW THIS LINE

5-12 If you're depositing a check into your account and want cash back, which type of endorsement would you use?

The restrictive endorsement tells what is to be done with the check. An example is writing <u>For Deposit Only</u> above your signature. The check can only be used as directed by the endorsement. No one can use your check in any other way. Don't write <u>For Deposit Only</u> on your check if you want to receive some of your deposit back in cash.

A special endorsement allows you to sign over to someone else a check that is written to you. You would sign your name and write your account number (if needed). Below this, you would write <u>Pay to the Order of</u> followed by the person's name. The person you name is the only one who can cash or deposit the check. This type of endorsement is not often used.

Making a Deposit

For each deposit you make, you'll need to fill out a deposit slip. See Figure 5-13. Give all the needed information. Sign the deposit slip if you want cash back from the deposit. Be sure to endorse any checks you deposit.

When you make a deposit, you will receive a receipt. Before you leave the bank, check this receipt. Make sure it lists the correct amount of your deposit. If you note a mistake, ask the teller to

5-13 This deposit slip contains all the information needed to make a deposit into this checking account.

correct it. Keep your receipt as a record of the deposit. Record the amount and date of the deposit in your checkbook register. Check all deposit receipts for the month against your statement.

Writing a Check

To write a check, fill in the spaces as indicated in Figure 5-14. Use dark, gel-type ink so nothing can be erased or altered. Write the number for the dollar amount close to the dollar sign on the check. This also prevents anyone from changing your check.

If you make a mistake, destroy the check and begin again. Do not make corrections on a check. Once you write a check, be sure to record the check number, amount, payee (person or business to whom you wrote the check), and date in your checkbook register. Subtract the amount from your current balance so you always know how much money is in your account.

Balancing Your Account

As you use your checking account, you will keep a record of all your transactions. The bank keeps a record, too. Comparing your records with those of the bank is called balancing your account. For

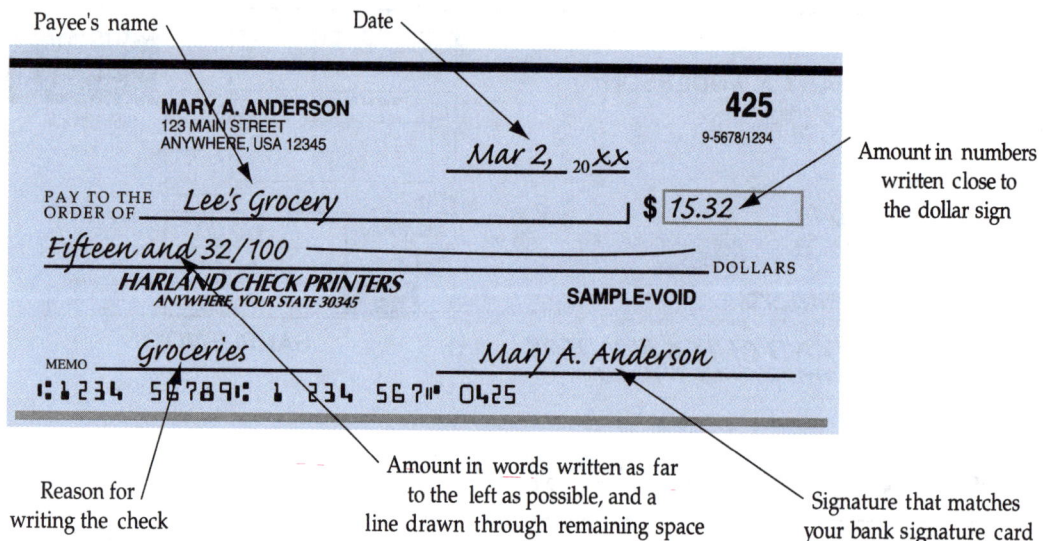

Payee's name — Date

MARY A. ANDERSON
123 MAIN STREET
ANYWHERE, USA 12345
425
9-5678/1234

Mar 2, 20XX

PAY TO THE ORDER OF   Lee's Grocery $ 15.32

Amount in numbers written close to the dollar sign

Fifteen and 32/100 ——— DOLLARS

HARLAND CHECK PRINTERS
ANYWHERE, YOUR STATE 30345   SAMPLE-VOID

MEMO   Groceries   Mary A. Anderson

⑈1234 567891⑈ 1 234 5671⑈ 0425

Reason for writing the check

Amount in words written as far to the left as possible, and a line drawn through remaining space

Signature that matches your bank signature card

5-14 Writing checks correctly takes a little practice, but it's a skill you can soon master.

this purpose, the bank sends statements that list all the activity in your account. These are usually sent monthly. This may depend on which type of account you have.

Note the opening and closing dates on your statement. All the transactions you made between these dates should be listed on the statement. This includes deposits and withdrawals, checks paid, ATM and debit card activity, and fees and other charges. See Figure 5-15. Your bank's statement may differ slightly from this sample. A personal banker can explain your bank's statement to you.

At first glance, your statement and checkbook register may not agree. Look at the date on the statement. This is the closing date, or the day the bank printed the statement. Transactions after this date are not reflected on your statement. Your register should be current. It should list all the transactions made.

To balance your account, you will need to follow several steps.

1. Account for all the items on your statement. Compare your receipts from deposits and ATM or debit cards to items on the statement. Place a checkmark in your register by each transaction that is on the statement and also in your register. Suppose you find transactions on your statement that are not in your register. (Some of these may be fees and other charges.) Enter these in your register. Make sure all the amounts match between the register and statement. Adjust your register as needed.

National Bank
Anytown, U.S.A.

ACCOUNT NUMBER
123-45-67-8
PAGE 1
NO. OF CHECKS 10

THIS STATEMENT DATE AND BALANCE		DEBITS AMOUNT	NUMBER	SERVICE CHARGE
3/31/XX	$48.73	$246.29	10	5.00

LAST STATEMENT DATE AND BALANCE		CREDITS AMOUNT	NUMBER	
2/28/XX	$50.02	$250.00	2	

STATEMENT OF ACCOUNT

Sarah Student
2647 Evergreen Drive
Anytown, U.S.A.

DAY	REF	CHECKS AND OTHER DEBITS AMT	REF	CHECKS AND OTHER DEBITS AMT	DEPOSITS AND OTHER CREDITS	DAILY BALANCE
3/2	488	15.32				34.70
3/4	489	25.00				9.70
3/9	490	5.25				4.45
3/11					130.00	134.45
3/15	ATM, National Bank	80.00				54.45
3/16	492	23.07				31.38
3/21	493	18.35				13.03
3/23					120.00	133.03
3/25	494	34.60				98.43
3/26	495	12.20				86.23
3/28	496	7.50				78.73
3/30	497	25.00				53.73
3/30		5.00		SERVICE CHARGE		48.73

5-15 A checking account statement is the bank's record of all the activity in your account during the statement period. Compare this with your checkbook register to make sure the two agree.

2. Next, turn to the balance worksheet on the back of your statement. See Figure 5-16 for a sample. If your statement doesn't have a balance worksheet, make your own using the figure as a guide. Write the closing balance shown on the statement in the space provided.

BALANCING WORKSHEET

CHECKS AND DEBITS OUTSTANDING
(Written but not shown on statement because not yet received by Bank.)

MONTH _March --_ , 20 _XX_

CLOSING BALANCE
shown on this statement $ _48.73_

ADD+

$ _125.00_

DEPOSITS made but not shown on statement because made or received after date of this statement.

TOTAL $ _173.73_

SUBTRACT –

CHECKS
OUTSTANDING .... $ _68.40_

BALANCE............... $ _105.33_

The above balance should be same as the up-to-date balance in your checkbook.

NO.		
498	28	40
499	15	00
ATM	25	00
TOTAL	68	40

5-16 The balancing worksheet on the back of your bank statement can seem a little tricky. It's just a step-by-step way to balance your account.

3. Find any deposits in your checkbook register that don't yet appear on your statement. These are the deposits without checkmarks in your register. List these deposits on the lines given.

4. List and total all the outstanding checks and ATM or debit card withdrawals or purchases in the column provided. Write this total in the space provided.

5. Add the deposits you listed in Step 3 to the closing balance. Write the total in the space provided.

6. Next, subtract the total you obtained in Step 4. This figure should match the final balance in your checkbook register. If not, go through all the steps again until you find the problem. When the statement and the register agree, the account is balanced.

Balancing your account is easiest when you keep careful records. Keep your checkbook register up-to-date. Be sure to balance your account each time you receive a statement. Waiting makes this much more difficult.

Managing Account Cards

When you open your account, you may receive an ATM card, which will let you use an automated teller machine (ATM). This machine lets you take money out of or put money into your account. ATM machines give you access to your account 24 hours a day.

If your bank offers an ATM card, it will also have an ATM machine. This is often outside the bank. Some banks own several machines in one town or city. These may be at convenient locations, such as stores, malls, and airports. Using an ATM machine owned by your bank is usually free. Your card will also work in most ATM machines owned by other banks. Both your bank and the other bank may charge you fees to use these machines.

To access your account using an ATM card, you need to know your personal identification number (PIN). This identifies your account. It is known by only you and the bank. Your PIN prevents others from using your ATM card to access your account. Even if your card is lost or stolen, no one can use it. For this reason, guard your PIN carefully. Do not tell this number to anyone or let anyone watch you enter it at the ATM machine. Do not write your PIN on the card or carry it in your wallet. Instead, memorize it or write it in a safe place where no one else can find it.

Another card that might come with your account is a debit card. This might also be called a check card. You can use this card to purchase goods and services. Your debit card comes with a PIN. In some places, you will need this PIN to make a purchase. In others, you can buy without the PIN.

When making purchases, the debit card is used much like a credit card. Also, instead of charging the purchase, the amount comes directly from your checking account. An advantage of the debit card is you can use it in many places that do not accept checks. This keeps you from having to carry large amounts of cash.

The debit card can also be used at an ATM machine when you enter the PIN. In fact, some banks no longer offer ATM cards because the debit card can be used in this way. Suppose your bank offers just a debit card. What if you don't want to use the card to make purchases? Ask your bank to set the debit limit at zero dollars. This will keep the card from being used in this way. Then, if the card is lost or stolen, no one can purchase items with the money in your checking account.

It's important to keep careful records of any transactions you make with an ATM or debit card. Record debit purchases in your checkbook register just as you would with a check. Don't forget to include in your register any fees or charges for using these cards. Keep your receipts to match against your bank statement as you balance your account. Call the bank if you note any errors.

Next, realize it's your job to know how much money is in your account. Do not use your card to make purchases your account can't cover. The fees charged for overdrawing your account are much like those for writing a bad check. They can affect your account in the same way.

Remember your budget when making purchases or taking cash from your account. Don't let your card influence you to make impulse buys or spend money you need for other items. See Figure 5-17. This can get you into trouble when it comes time to pay your bills.

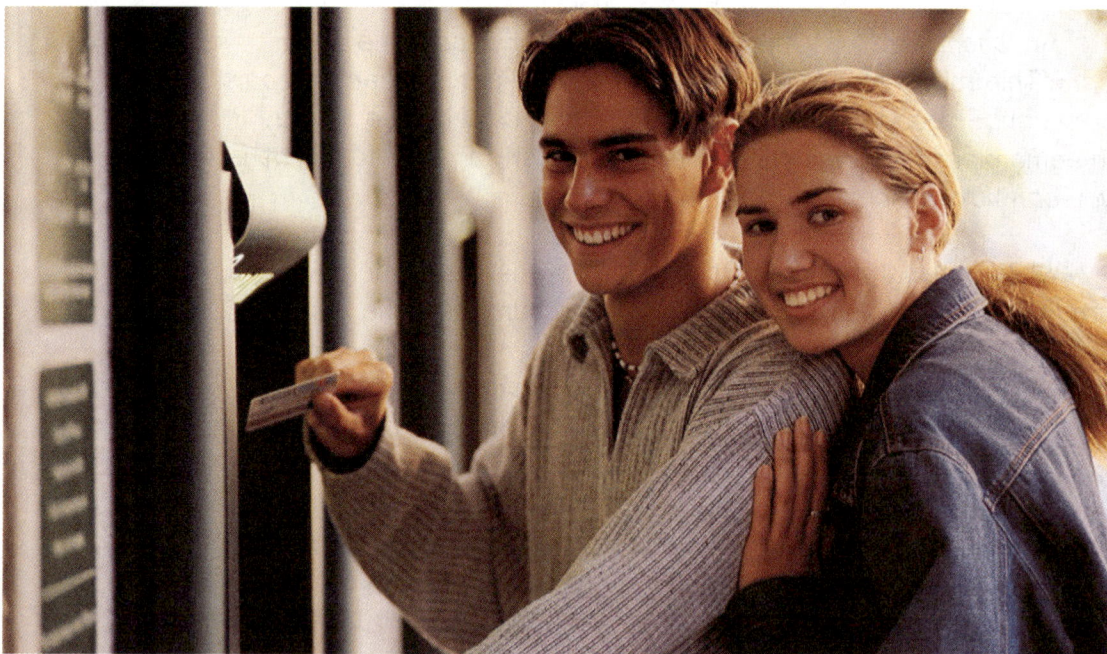

5-17 Most of the time, the money you withdraw from an ATM machine should be money you included in your budget. Avoid using the ATM to make impulse purchases.

Other Check-Cashing Options

For various reasons, some teens have never used a bank. They may not feel comfortable with the idea of banking. These teens may turn to check-cashing services or currency exchanges. These businesses operate for a profit. Most often they are found in large towns and cities. Their goal is to make money from cashing checks for you. Each transaction you make at one of these businesses will cost you.

Suppose you need to cash your paycheck every week. If you have a bank account, you can cash checks at the bank for no charge. At a check-cashing service or currency exchange, you will pay a fee to cash each check. This fee is often several dollars. It is set by the business and depends on the amount of your check. You'll pay a larger fee for cashing a larger check. During a year, you could pay more than a hundred dollars in these fees. That's quite a bit of money that could go to other items on your budget.

Other services these businesses provide are also costly. If you don't have a checking account, you may need to buy money orders to pay your bills. A money order is a piece of paper on which the issuer orders a specific amount to be paid to the payee. (The issuer is the bank, post office, or business that sells the money order. The payee is the person or company to whom the money order is written.) You pay the issuer to create the money order for you. You can send the money order to the payee just as if it were a check.

You must pay a service charge for each money order you buy. If you need many money orders, these fees add up quickly. With a checking account, the fee per check (if any) is lower than this service fee. Over time, you could save a lot of money by using checks to pay your bills.

If you've been using currency exchanges or check-cashing services often, you might reconsider. Visit a few banks and learn about the services they offer. Find out how much time and money you would save by opening an account. This can help you decide whether a checking account is a good option for you.

Major Points

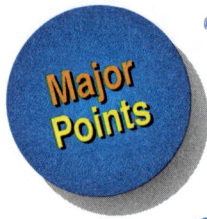

☞ Wise use of credit can help you build financial security and protect the well-being of yourself and your baby. Credit offers the benefit of buying now and paying later. However, credit costs money and misusing it carries serious consequences.

☞ Two kinds of consumer credit are sales credit and cash credit. You can use sales credit through a store or credit card to buy goods and services. You can use cash credit in the form of a loan to buy a car, pay for college, or meet other long-term financial goals.

☞ The cost of credit depends on how much you use, what rate of interest is charged, and how long you take to repay. Consider these factors each time you choose whether to use credit for a particular purchase.

☞ Credit contracts and agreements are the papers you sign when you apply for and use credit. They define the legal responsibilities of both the creditor and the borrower. Be sure you understand all the terms in a credit contract before you sign it.

☞ Several laws protect you when you use credit. Learn what protections these laws offer so you can be sure your rights are honored.

☞ Managing credit takes self-control. When used wisely, credit can be a good money management tool. Risky uses of credit can lead to trouble, though. If credit problems develop, deal with them promptly. Consider seeking reliable credit counseling.

☞ Insurance is an agreement between you and an insurance company to share the risks of financial loss. You can insure your car, home, belongings, life, and health to protect your family from loss if a crisis occurs.

☞ Personal bank accounts are a useful financial tool. A savings account is a safe place to store your money and let it earn interest. A checking account offers a convenient way to buy goods and services, pay bills, and keep your money safe. To manage these accounts well, you need to learn how to handle financial transactions.

Chapter 6
Planning for
the Future

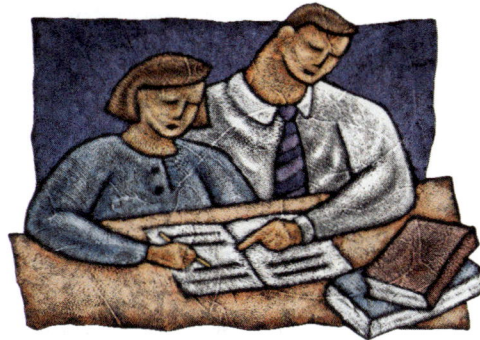

By the time your baby arrives, you will probably have formed some kind of plan about how you will financially support her for now. Your family and the baby's father may help you with money. You may have a part-time job to help pay the bills. Especially at first, you may also receive some type of public assistance. This might be through the Temporary Assistance for Needy Families Bureau (TANF). Public aid can help you get on your feet and care for your child.

Even if you have a workable plan for right now, you need to plan for the future. You will have to support your child until she's an adult. You'll want to be able to meet her basic needs. Current laws limit how long you can receive public aid. In many states, there is a five-year lifetime limit. This means if you start getting aid today, your benefits will end in five years. You won't be eligible for any more help from the public aid system. In some states, there may be an exception to this rule. Ask your caseworker.

This means you have only a few years to prepare to fully support your child. It's wise to use this time to plan and prepare for the future. Right now, you may qualify to receive assistance with food and housing, as well as cash payments. You may also be able to get help with school tuition, child care, and job training. Public aid programs vary from state to state. Ask a caseworker at your local public aid office what help you might be able to receive.

You may not want to be on public aid, but accepting all this help now can enable you to be financially independent in the future. When you begin to earn your own income, you will pay taxes on your income that will help others in need.

Now is the time to plan for your future. What is your life like now? What do you want to be different five to ten years from now? What kind of life do you want to create for yourself and your baby? Answering these questions will help you decide what goals to set. This chapter will guide you through making career decisions and setting the goals needed to get there.

What Does the Future Hold?

Before you begin to plan your future, take a look at your present situation. Where are you now, and what is going on in your life? Are you going to school? Have you ever had a job? Are you working now? What job training or experience have you had? What public aid are you receiving? Do you qualify for more? What support do you have from the baby's father and his family, as well as your family and friends?

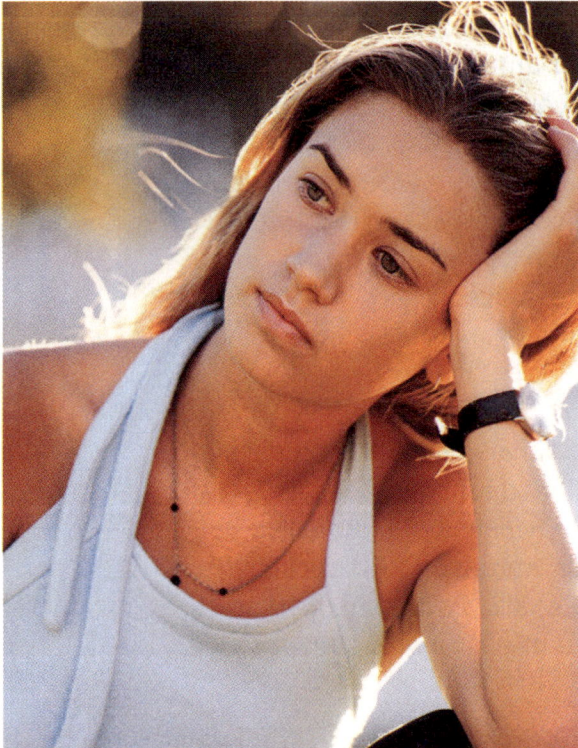

With a clear picture of where you are right now, you can start planning what you want the future to hold. Imagine yourself in a year, three years, and five years. See Figure 6-1. In what ways do you want your life to remain the same? How do you want it to be different? What changes do you hope to make? Your answers to these questions can help you set realistic goals for the future.

One of your first goals will be to prepare to enter the world of work. You will need a job to become

6-1 It's important to take some time to think about your life and make plans for the future.

financially independent and pay your expenses. It may be necessary to start at a low-paying job. You may earn only the minimum wage. This is the lowest hourly wage employers are allowed to pay. The amount is set by law and adjusted from time to time. Your first job may not pay all your expenses, but the experience you gain will help you get a better job in the future.

As a teen parent, your immediate focus may be finding a job—any job that will help pay your bills. Taking care of yourself and a child costs money. You might even have to take a job you don't like just to earn money or meet the work requirements for TANF. It is good to be concerned about what you will do right now to meet your expenses. This shows you are responsible.

On the other hand, it's also good to think about the future and what career you'd like to pursue. You need to start thinking about this now because it requires a plan. Suppose you want to be a teacher. This will take planning and a lot of hard work. You must first finish high school. Then you must go to college to earn a teaching degree. It will mean a few more years of school. Since reaching this goal will take some time, it's best to start planning now.

Being a teen parent doesn't mean your dreams can't come true. However, you may have to be more determined and work harder than your friends who aren't parents. It may take you longer to reach your goals than if you weren't a parent. This is because your child needs so much of your time, energy, and attention. See Figure 6-2. Don't give up, though. You can do it!

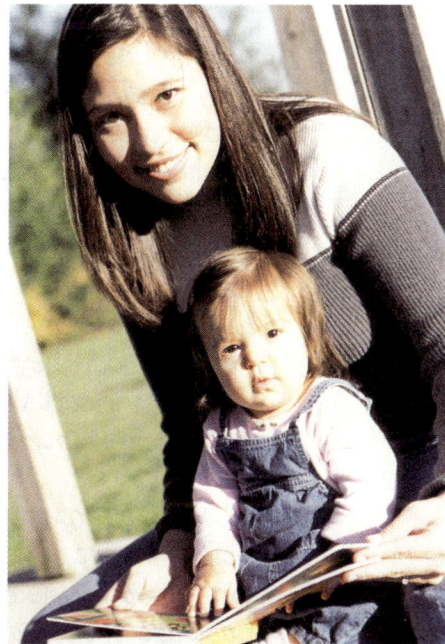

6-2 Being a parent is a full-time job! Your child needs love, guidance, and physical care.

Exploring Career Options

What do you want to be? At first, this question can seem intimidating. You may not have any idea what career you want to pursue. You may not know what jobs are available in different fields.

You may not have thought about what you'd be good at or what you'd like to do. To make the best career choice, you will want to explore your options.

This means doing some research about careers. As you investigate career fields, think about how each might suit you. For each field that interests you, take notes on the jobs available. What are the duties, requirements, and pay? Keep these notes to compare fields and determine what's best for you. You can turn to many sources to learn more about different careers.

Counselors, Teachers, and Caseworkers

A guidance counselor can help you explore careers. This person has special training to advise you in this area. He or she may be able to arrange for you to take some tests to learn more about yourself. These tests will identify your strengths, weaknesses, and skills. They can teach you about your personality and interests. Your counselor can direct you to other career-related resources you can explore.

Teachers or caseworkers can often guide you through career choices, too. They may know about job opportunities and how to prepare for certain types of work. Ask them to direct you to other career information you may need.

These professionals can be valuable contacts for you. They can help you sort out your thoughts about a career. It's your choice, but these people can help talk you through it. They may know of job openings that might interest you. They can often serve as references for you, both now and in the future.

Career Information Guides

The U.S. Department of Labor publishes three main career information guides. These guides offer detailed information about job and career choices. You can find these guides in your school or public library. They are also online. Spending some time with each guide can help you decide what type of work would be right for you.

- ☛ The <u>Occupational Outlook Handbook</u> describes more than 250 types of jobs. Use it to look up a certain job or see what types of jobs interest you. This guide also tells what education or training you'll need for a job and what pay to expect.

- ☛ The <u>Guide for Occupational Exploration</u> can help you learn about yourself and decide what type of career you want. It can help you explore your personality, interests, and skills. This guide also lists 12 basic career areas. For each area, it describes the skills and traits workers need. Look up the career area that interests you to see if it would be a good match for you.

- ☛ The Occupational Information Network, called O*NET, is an online resource at **www.onetcenter.org**. Use it to explore careers, trends, and needed job skills. It also helps you check your abilities and career interests.

Other Library Resources

Both school and public libraries have more resources you can use to learn about careers. Many libraries have set up special sections for employment resources. In others, it may take a bit more looking to find what you want. You may find books, newspapers, journals, and magazines on jobs and careers to be helpful. The library might also have brochures from local job training programs. Specific resources will vary from one library to another. Take some time to learn what your libraries have to offer. If you need help, be sure to ask the library staff.

Internet

Go online to investigate careers that interest you. See Figure 6-3. If you can't access the Internet at

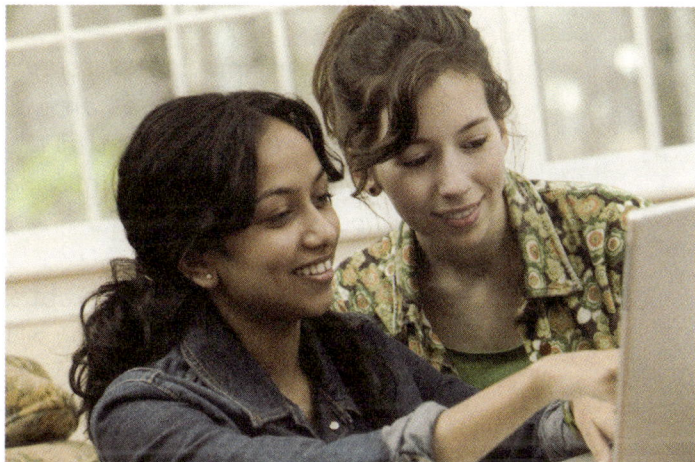

6-3 The Internet can be a valuable resource as you research career fields.

home, use the connection at your public library, school, or community center. If you aren't comfortable using the Internet, maybe a counselor, teacher, or friend can guide you.

Online information can include guides to resumes, interviews, job success, and other related topics. Some job training programs and courses are even offered online for credit. This may be a good idea for you if you can go online at home. Ask a counselor or teacher to help you evaluate these courses before you sign up. This will help you avoid wasting your time or money.

Choosing a Career Field

After doing research, you will likely find several job opportunities in fields that interest you. Now it's time to narrow it down to one or two fields you might want to pursue. Take some time to figure out what you want from a job besides a paycheck. You want to choose the career field that will be the most satisfying for you.

How does the career you're considering fit with your values? What is really important to you? What do you want to do with your life? What type of work would you feel proud to do? The answers to these questions will reveal some of your values about work. Choose a career that goes well with your values. If your job clashes with your values, you'll probably soon find yourself unhappy.

Your skills are important, too. A job will be most satisfying when you can do it well. What are your strongest skills? What jobs would help you make the most of these skills? What skills might you need to develop more before entering your chosen career field? How could you build these skills?

Next, think about your interests. What do you like to do? No matter what career you pick, you will spend a good part of your future working. Life will be sweeter if you find work you like and feel good about doing. See Figure 6-4 for a checklist that can help you identify types of work that may suit you.

Job Interest Checklist

I like to work with the following (check all that apply):

❑ people	❑ ideas	❑ cars
❑ animals	❑ plants	❑ art materials
❑ numbers	❑ tools	❑ electronic equipment
❑ computers	❑ books	❑ other: _____
❑ children	❑ food	❑ other: _____

Work areas that interest me include the following (check all that apply):

❑ accounting	❑ cosmetology	❑ public safety
❑ acting	❑ education	❑ sales
❑ advertising	❑ food service	❑ science
❑ agriculture/farming	❑ health services	❑ social services
❑ armed forces	❑ journalism	❑ sports
❑ art/graphic design	❑ law	❑ other: _____
❑ child care	❑ office work	❑ other: _____
❑ computer careers	❑ politics	❑ other: _____

6-4   What type of work interests you?

Finally, learn what the current job trends are in your chosen field. You don't want to prepare for a career in which job opportunities are limited. This would make it hard for you to find work. Look for a career that is expanding and offers many job opportunities.

Look into job trends and predictions in the fields that interest you. Contact the U.S. Department of Labor to learn more. You can also find this information in career books and Web sites. Talking to someone in the field might give you more insight about what the career really involves.

Compare your notes on all the career areas you're still considering. Seek any additional information you need before making your choice. When you have all the information you need, it's time to choose the career field you think will suit you best. Figure 6-5 lists jobs in various career fields that seem to be growing quickly.

Some Job Options to Consider

Agriculture, Food, and Natural Resources
❖ pet shop operator, golf course groundskeeper, meat cutter, water-quality monitor

Architecture and Construction
❖ carpenter, interior decorator, painter, cost estimator, carpet installer

Arts, Audio/Video Technology, and Communications
❖ make-up artist, set designer, line repairer/installer, control room technician

Business Management and Administration
❖ payroll clerk, order processor, demonstrator, human resources assistant

Education and Training
❖ teacher's aid, preschool assistant, social worker, parent educator, coach

Finance
❖ bank teller, data processor, sales agent, processing clerk, credit report provider

Government and Public Administration
❖ court reporter, census taker, legal aide, program assistant, city clerk

Health Science
❖ lab technician, foodservice worker, medical biller, records assistant, paramedic

Hospitality and Tourism
❖ tour guide, receptionist, travel coordinator, banquet server, housekeeper

Human Services
❖ childcare worker, hairstylist, personal trainer, coordinator of volunteers

Information Technology
❖ programmer, software tester, production assistant, database associate

Law, Public Safety, Corrections, and Security
❖ rescue worker, dispatcher, firefighter, park ranger, control center operator

Manufacturing
❖ safety technician, materials mover, purchasing agent, machine operator

Marketing
❖ sales representative, stock clerk, customer service specialist, copywriter

Science, Technology, Engineering, and Mathematics
❖ science teacher, automotive specialist, lab technician, technical writer

Transportation, Distribution, and Logistics
❖ shipping clerk, truck driver, aircraft cargo handler, dispatcher, warehouse clerk

6-5 These jobs are currently experiencing rapid growth. Workers can often find job opportunities in these career fields.

Setting Career Goals

Once you've chosen a career field, it's time to set career goals. Your main long-term goal is to work in your chosen field. To reach this goal, you will have to set and reach many smaller goals along the way. You want your goals to be steps on the path toward reaching your long-term goal. These steps should begin today and carry you through until you are working in the job of your choice.

As you set career goals, there are many factors to consider. The following questions can help you explore what these goals should be:

☞ What is required before I can work in this career field? You may need a set type and amount of education or training. A license or certificate might be required. You may need to gain experience in a related entry-level or part-time job first. Each of these requirements can be one of your mid-term or long-term goals.

☞ Are there tasks I must complete before I can start to meet these requirements? For example, to go to college, you must first earn a high school diploma or a GED. You might need to take classes or training before you earn your license or certificate. Each task will be a mid-term or short-term goal.

☞ What can I do right now to advance my long-term career goals? If you're in high school, your academic performance may be a key part of your long-term career goal. This is especially true for competitive career fields. Doing well at your part-time job is a way to earn valuable references for future jobs. Volunteer work in your career field can help build your resume. Keeping the larger picture in mind can help you get through times when your long-term goal seems unreachable.

Considering these questions can help you set realistic career goals. Each time you meet a short- or mid-term goal, you will be one step closer to the job of your choice. Always keep the larger picture in mind. This can help you get through times when your long-term goal seems unreachable. (If you need more information on how to set goals, see another title in this series, Understanding Your Changing Life.)

Getting the Training and Education You Need

Generally, the more education and job-related training you have, the better job opportunities you will have in the years ahead. Education and training can help you learn more about the career field you want to enter. You can gain the skills employers in the field value. This will make you more desirable as an employee.

Once you've set career goals, you know what education and training you will need to reach these goals. You can begin to plan how you will obtain this education or training. Most jobs require at least a high school diploma or GED. This should be a top priority, because it will open many doors for you. Many jobs require even more education and training than high school or the GED. You might need to enroll in school-to-work programs, occupational training, or college to become qualified to work in your chosen career.

Finishing High School

Completing your high school education is important no matter what type of career you want. See Figure 6-6. It can be difficult to return to school when you have a baby. Parenting will demand a lot from you, and it can be hard to juggle both the roles of parent and student.

Having a baby makes your education even more important, though. You need to become able to support yourself and your child. This takes a lot of money. By finishing high school, you can qualify for a job that will help you earn more money. Both you and your child will benefit.

You have a legal right to complete your high school education. No one can keep you from doing that. Federal laws make it illegal for schools to discriminate on the basis of gender. Since pregnancy happens only to women, it is seen as gender discrimination to have different rules for students who are pregnant or who have given birth. Your state may have more laws that protect your rights to an education.

In most states, you must be allowed to attend school until you give birth. After your baby is born, you must be allowed to return to this same school if you choose. Laws do vary from state to state. Find out what your state's laws say about this. Your teacher or counselor should know the laws and your school's policies.

With your rights come responsibilities. You are expected to attend school regularly. Try not to miss school unless you are ill. If you are ill, have your doctor write a note explaining the absence. Try to keep up with your schoolwork. Avoid making appointments during school hours if possible. Work with your teachers to make up any work you miss. Finally, you have the responsibility to return to school as soon as possible after having your baby.

6-6   Concentrating on your studies may seem difficult now, but it will pay off later in increased job opportunities.

Some school districts have programs designed especially for pregnant and parenting teens. These might be special classes, programs, or even separate schools for pregnant and parenting teens. Find out what your district offers. Then you can decide if these programs would be best for you.

Programs for pregnant and parenting teens do have some benefits. First, you may find comfort in the support of peers who are also pregnant or parenting. Second, these programs are designed to meet your unique needs as a teen parent or parent-to-be. See Figure 6-7. Ask these questions if you're thinking about switching to one of these alternative programs.

You might prefer to stay in your own school with your friends. This might be more familiar to you. In most states, the decision must be yours. This means no one can force you to be in an alternative program. You can decide what will best meet your needs.

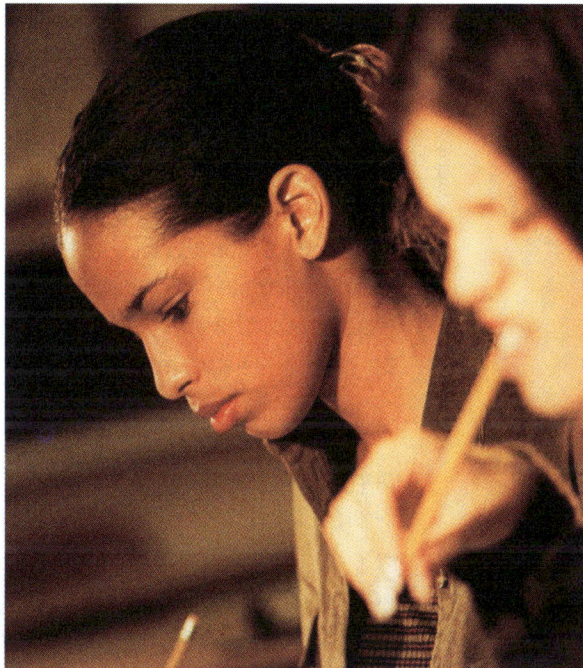

Graduation Versus GED

Graduating is one way to complete your high school education. A second way is to earn your general equivalency diploma (GED). You could earn this diploma through the General Education Development program. In this program, you would take classes to prepare for the GED test. When you pass this test, you would earn your diploma. The test is designed to show whether you've mastered the material taught in high schools. Refer to Chapter 1 to review what the GED is or how it works.

Most schools and employers see the GED as equal to high school graduation. With a GED, you can enter college, a career or technical school, or other training programs. For some students, earning the GED is the best way to earn a diploma. Others find they gain more from completing high school and participating in school activities. The choice is yours.

Your teachers, counselor, or school district office should be able to tell you more about getting a GED. They can tell you when and where the classes are held. Ask if there's an age requirement or if a fee applies. Before you begin these classes, be sure you can give the time and energy needed to study and prepare for the exam.

Is an Alternative School or Program for Me?

If your school district has a special school or program for pregnant and parenting teens, you might consider transferring. Before you do, however, you should ask some important questions.

* If I transfer in the middle of a term, does the new program offer the same classes I currently have? If not, will I have to repeat those classes?

* Will I have to make up work if there's a difference between my old classes and my new ones?

* What will happen to my grade point average and credits if I transfer? Will I still graduate on time?

* Could I re-enroll in my regular program or school? How would I do this?

Adapted with permission from the Illinois Caucus on Adolescent Health

6-7 Consider these questions carefully when evaluating an alternative school program.

Completing your high school education is important. This is true whether you choose to graduate or earn the GED. Start planning right away—you don't want to waste any time in reaching this goal.

School-to-Work Programs

Find out if there is a program in your area that prepares students for the workplace. These programs are often called school-to-work programs. They offer work-based learning for high school students. If you enter this type of program, you will gain the experience you will need for employment. The program will prepare you for your first job in a high-skill, high-wage field. It may open the door to further education, too.

School-to-work programs take you from full-time student to full-time worker. They combine work experience and classroom learning. Most also provide pay. These programs can introduce you to a variety of career paths. You can choose the one that best matches your skills and interests.

When you enter a school-to-work program, you are assigned a mentor at the worksite. This person will guide you through the workplace. Through this experience, you will also learn more about the attitudes and behaviors needed to succeed on the job. After you complete this type of program, you should be able to enter the workforce right away.

To find out about work-based learning in your area, ask at your school. You also can contact the local school board or state department of education to learn more.

Internships

You might also want to look into an internship. This program offers short-term work and learning experience in a career field. Its purpose is to introduce you to the field. Some internships are paid. Others are done on a volunteer basis.

The key to getting an internship is knowing what's available. Your school counselor may know of some openings. You can also look for <u>Peterson's Guide to Internships</u> at your school or public library. This yearly guide describes internships in 22 career fields. The Internet can be a good source of up-to-date information about internships.

Apprenticeships

An apprenticeship combines on-the-job training and classroom learning. It helps people learn the highly specialized skills they need to work in the craft or trade industries. A youth apprenticeship is available to high school students. It offers basic job training and classroom work. A registered apprenticeship requires a high school diploma or GED. It is much more advanced.

When you research your chosen career, find out if apprenticeships are offered or required in this field. About 350 apprenticeship programs are registered with the Bureau of Apprenticeship and Training (BAT). This is a division of the U.S. Department of Labor. You can contact the nearest state or regional BAT office to learn more.

Occupational Training

Occupational training will prepare you to work in a certain field. This type of training is valuable if you know what you want to do. You can find occupational training in many places. It may be offered by private schools, community colleges, vocational schools, or employer-sponsored programs.

Occupational training is offered in a wide variety of fields. You could study to become a dental or medical assistant, office worker, or court reporter. You might become a baker, hair stylist, automotive technician, truck driver, woodworker, or computer repair person. Occupational training can prepare you for good jobs in many fields.

Suppose occupational training is required or suggested for your field. How do you get started? Talk to your guidance counselor, teacher, or a trusted adult. You can also look online to see what training programs are available. Find out what the requirements are to enroll in programs that interest you. You may need a high school diploma or GED. Work experience may be required. You'll need to meet the requirements before you can enroll in the program.

Before you enroll in any occupational training, investigate the program thoroughly so you know what to expect. Use the questions in Figure 6-8 to help you choose a training program.

Choosing a Training School or Program

The following questions may help you evaluate training schools and programs.

❖ What will the training cost? What scholarships or other assistance might I be qualified to receive?

❖ What courses are offered and what skills will I learn?

❖ What entrance requirements must I meet?

❖ How long will it take to complete the program or course of study? How much study time will I need to give it day-by-day outside of class?

❖ What are the attendance and performance requirements for completing the course or training?

❖ Who will teach the courses or trainings and what are their qualifications?

❖ What is the average class size?

❖ Are facilities and equipment up-to-date and adequate for the number of students?

❖ How many of the students are successfully employed after finishing courses and programs of study?

❖ What job search assistance can the program or school provide?

❖ Is the school or program licensed or accredited by industry or educational agencies?

❖ Do employers and former students recommend the school or program?

❖ What will I be qualified to do when I have completed the training? Will I receive a degree, license, or certification?

6-8 If you choose a reputable training program, occupational training can prepare you for a rewarding career.

College

Once you complete high school, you may want to think about college. Many high-paying jobs will require you to have a college degree. It is an advantage in almost all careers. Even a job that doesn't require a degree may pay you more if you have one. A college degree may also open more job opportunities to you in the future.

Does your chosen career require a degree? If so, what type of degree will you need? Associate degrees are offered in many career fields at community or junior colleges. It usually takes two years of study to earn this degree. In a four-year college program, you can earn a bachelor's degree. Some jobs require a graduate degree. This type of degree takes even more school after the bachelor's degree.

It might be best to start at a community or junior college. These schools are smaller and offer more personal attention than large colleges. They also cost less than a four-year university. After two years, you can often transfer your credits to a four-year school if you wish. By then, you would have experience with college life and classes. This would help you feel more confident at a four-year school where the classes are often much larger. You will have learned where and how to seek help when you need it.

Colleges differ greatly. There are many factors to think about when you are making this choice. First, you need to choose a school that offers the course of study you want. You'll also want to find out what facilities the campus has to offer. These might include a library, student center, and computer labs. Next, check out the academic reputation of the school. You want to pick a school with a solid reputation. Class size can be important, too.

Today, many colleges welcome young parents, both married and single. Is the school you're looking at one of these? Find out if the school offers any special programs for parenting students. Would you qualify for these programs? How would this make college easier for you?

When choosing a school, you'll also want to think about living arrangements. If you go to a school near home, could you and your child live with your family while you're in school? This would be a great help, because you could save the money you would have spent for room and board. You might also receive more daily support and help from your family if you live with them. For these reasons, you might pick a school that is close so you could live at home.

If you're going away to school, find out what housing the school offers for students who are also parents. If there is no housing on campus for families, what housing is available in the community?

Can you find affordable housing? If you're a single parent, perhaps you could find a roommate who also has a child. This would let you split the costs and find some support.

Housing costs are only one type of cost related to college. Before you enroll, find out the total cost of tuition, fees, books, and other expenses. At first, this figure can seem overwhelming. You'll need to develop a plan to meet these costs.

Many students receive financial aid from their schools. This aid comes in many forms. You might qualify for a grant. This is federal, state, or local money given to low-income students to help them pay for college. You do not have to repay a grant.

Another option might be a scholarship. This is a special award that pays all or part of college tuition and other costs. It doesn't have to be repaid. There are thousands of scholarships available from many sources. To find out what you might qualify for, you will need to do some research. Online sources may provide some of the most up-to-date information. Your school counselor may have some information, too.

You may be able to earn a scholarship with good grades or special talents you've shown in high school. Some scholarships are for single parents who want to go to college. See Figure 6-9. Others may be based on what field you're going into or where you come from.

Find out if your college has a work-study program. This program would connect you with a job on campus. One advantage of work-study is that any money you earn from this job won't count as income when you apply for financial

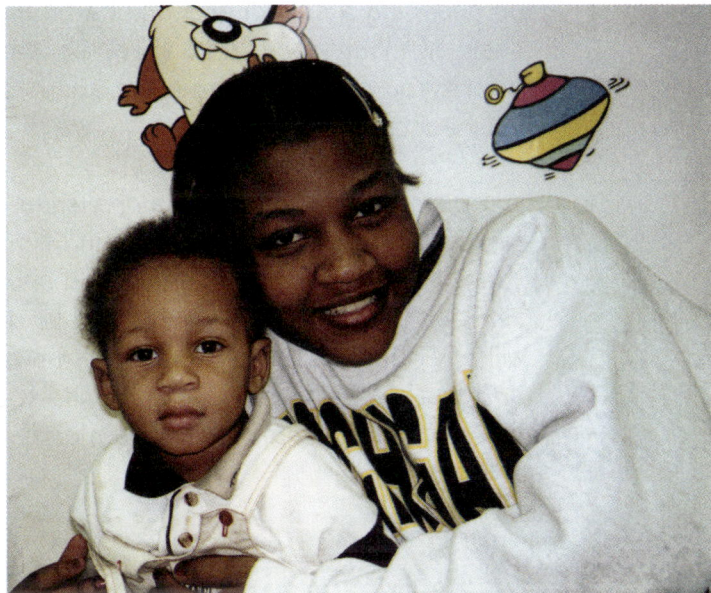

6-9   With a little research, you may be able to find scholarships designed for young parents who want to go to college.

aid the following year. If you have another type of job, your earnings would count against you when applying for financial aid. This might make you less eligible for aid the next year.

Finally, you can take out loans to pay for college. These loans are available from many sources. Once you leave school, you must repay the loans you take. For some students, borrowing this money is the only way to make college a reality. They view repaying loans after college a small price to pay for their higher earning power.

Look for a loan with a low interest rate. This will lower the amount you must repay. Be careful not to borrow more than you absolutely need. A large debt can cause money problems after you leave school.

Also, be careful to budget your financial aid or loan money carefully so it will last you a full semester. When you get your check at the first of the semester, it can be tempting to overspend. This will only lead you to serious problems later in the semester. Budget this money carefully to meet your expenses all semester long.

To learn more about colleges, ask a teacher or counselor. The Internet is an outstanding source of information. You can find tips on choosing a school and finding financial aid. Many schools have their own Web sites. Visit these to learn more about what a school offers. You can also read more about colleges and universities at your school or public library.

Going to college will be a challenge. Juggling all your responsibilities will be tough. You'll have to find time to attend classes, care for your child, study, and do household chores. You may also have a part-time job to help pay the bills. It will be difficult, but a college degree will pay off in better job opportunities and higher earnings. It will also add to the quality of life for you and your child. If you want it enough, you can work to make this dream come true. The power lies in you.

Preparing for a Job Search

Before you even begin to look for a job, you can take steps to prepare yourself for the world of work. You can start by improving your basic life skills. These are the skills you need to manage your life, finances, and home. You also can build the job-related skills you'll need to do your job well. Begin to investigate child care options, so you will know where to look when you find employment.

You may be able to work on some of these things while you're in school or training. You can also look into a job-readiness program. This is a program designed to help you move smoothly into the workforce. As you prepare to look for a job, it is important to consider what employers want in an employee.

What Makes a Good Employee?

Employers are looking for employees who will fit into the workplace. They want workers who can do the job they are hired to do. These employees have the personal characteristics that employers desire. They have the skills and training needed to perform well on the job.

Personal Characteristics

Put yourself in an employer's shoes for a moment. When hiring a new worker, what personal characteristics would appeal to you? Certain qualities are needed in all jobs. See Figure 6-10. Which of these traits would you want in an employee? What type of person would you want to represent your business or organization?

Employers want someone with a strong work ethic. A work ethic is a standard of conduct and values for job performance. A good employee will work hard and strive to perform at a high level. Employers also want workers who have a strong sense about what actions are right and wrong for the workplace. These workers will be honest and reliable.

The ability to get along with others is one of the most important traits employers want. It is essential for workers to get along with their supervisors, coworkers, and customers. This helps a business or organization run smoothly. Someone who can't get along with others will have trouble keeping a job.

What Do Employers Want from Workers?

Personal Traits	Related Employee Actions
Positive attitude	❖ wants to work ❖ shows an interest in doing the job well and advancing
Reliability	❖ comes to work every scheduled work day
Promptness	❖ arrives at work on time
Neat, clean appearance	❖ dresses appropriately for the job ❖ appears clean and well groomed for work
Honesty	❖ can be trusted
People skills	❖ works well with others and fits into the workplace ❖ pleases customers
Communication skills	❖ talks easily with boss and coworkers ❖ expresses ideas clearly
Strong work ethic	❖ looks for work to do without being told ❖ works hard even when no one is watching
Self-control	❖ expresses feelings appropriately and controls temper ❖ accepts direction and criticism

6-10 How many of these traits do you possess? How can you gain the others?

Attitude and image matter, too. Employers want pleasant workers who show a positive outlook on life. They want people who can make the best of a situation. Employees represent the company or agency that employs them. It is important for workers to come to work clean, neat, and dressed to fit the job. A sense of self-esteem and confidence should show in the way they carry themselves.

Now consider your own personality. How would you describe yourself? If you were an employer, would you hire you? Learn to make the most of your positive characteristics when you are job-hunting. Take some time to improve in areas where you may be lacking. This will make you better prepared when you start looking for work.

Skills and Qualifications

Employers want to hire someone who is qualified to do the job. They will want to know about your qualifications when you apply for a job. The exact qualifications an employer will seek depend on the job. They may include some of the following:

☞ education

☞ training

☞ previous work experience

☞ certifications or licenses

☞ awards or recognition you've received

☞ activities you've participated in that relate to the job

☞ other experiences that make you competent to work in this field

Your life experiences may help you qualify for a job. Think about what you've done at school, the workplace, and home. What have you learned that would make you a good employee? Use Figure 6-11

Assessing Your Qualifications

You can use the following questions to help you explore your qualifications for employment:

❖ How many years of school have I completed?

❖ What awards or recognition did I receive in school?

❖ What are my plans for continuing my education?

❖ What jobs have I already had?

❖ What responsibilities did I have at each job?

❖ What responsibilities do I have at home?

❖ How has the job of parenting helped me prepare for work outside the home?

❖ What are five things I do very well?

❖ What are/were my three favorite school activities?

❖ What are/were my three favorite subjects in school?

❖ What are five personality traits an employer would like about me?

❖ What are five areas in which I need to improve in order to do well on the job?

6-11 As you prepare for your job search, think about your qualifications and how you will present these to potential employers.

to explore your job qualifications. Think of ways to tell an employer how what you've learned as a student or worker has prepared you for the job you seek. This matters most when you have qualifications that wouldn't be obvious to the employer.

You must also have the skills that will enable you to do a job well. In each job, there are specific skills you need to do the work asked of you. For instance, if you're a salesclerk, you may need to use a cash register. If you want to work as a cook, you need the skills to prepare certain dishes. The job description can tell you what specific skills the employer wants you to have. If you're unsure, you can ask the employer what skills you need when you interview for the job.

No matter what job you have, you will need basic skills. These include reading, writing, math, speaking, and listening. Employers expect you to bring these skills to the job. To succeed on the job, you will also need to know how to think, solve problems, and make decisions. Employers also want to be sure you can make the best use of resources such as time, materials, and space.

Job Readiness Programs

Stepping into the workforce for the first time takes courage, determination, and help. A job readiness program can help you take the beginning steps toward full-time work. This is a short-term program designed to prepare you for the world of work. Employers are often involved in these programs. Their goal is to bring people into jobs that provide benefits and chances to advance.

Job readiness programs can help you gain soft skills. These are skills that will help you manage your life so you can hold a full-time job. Soft skills include the abilities to budget and manage money, to care for your baby and yourself, and to manage your home and time. By mastering these skills, you can focus on finding and succeeding at a full-time job.

Some of the needs a job readiness program might help you meet include the following:

- clothes for interviews and work
- finding and paying for reliable child care

- ☛ finding health care and paying medical costs
- ☛ arranging and paying for transportation
- ☛ support services while you search for, and become established in, a job

Job readiness programs also help you build the job skills you will need. You may receive training in good work habits, coping skills, and job search skills. Job readiness classes will introduce you to appropriate workplace behavior. They may also offer follow-up appointments after you're hired to help you keep your job and get ahead.

If you're interested in this type of program, find out if there is a program near you. A teacher, counselor, or caseworker might be able to refer you to one. You can also contact your state or local department of health and human services. In addition, some of these programs have Web sites you can visit.

Personal Preparations

To prepare for a full-time job, you will need to consider how you will handle some of your personal issues. Before taking a job, you will need to arrange for child care, clothes for the workplace, and transportation. You will also want to find ways to pay work-related expenses. In some cases, people who leave welfare for work lose some of their benefits. If this is the case, your expenses may increase. Eventually, the money you earn should more than make up the difference. Still, it can be difficult when you're just getting started.

You can find out rates and schedules for cabs, trains, and busses in your area prior to looking for a job. When you interview for jobs, ask about transportation to and from work. You may be able to join a car pool, which could save you money. With all this information, you'll be prepared to solve your transportation problem.

Look for ways to make up for any benefits you receive now that may be reduced or stopped when you're employed. Your caseworker can often help you with this. Be sure to ask about

Earned Income Tax Credit, which can be a great help to you. This tax credit is actually a wage supplement. You receive it from the Internal Revenue Service (IRS) after the tax-filing season. Workers with children may be able to use the Advance Payment Option. Then, part of the credit is added to each paycheck. The remainder comes in a lump sum at the end of the year. Check with the IRS to see if you qualify for this type of tax credit.

Clothes for work and for job interviews can be a problem for first-time employees. Finding and paying for appropriate clothing can be a challenge. You may be able to find help from some agencies in your community. In some areas, the social services office has a program that provides a one-time clothing stipend to help clients with clothing for interviews and jobs. Your community may have an organization that provides business clothing to women who are seeking work for the first time. These may require a referral from your caseworker. Consignment shops, resale clothing stores, and garage sales may be other ways to buy the clothing you need at the lowest prices.

This may sound like a lot of thinking and planning. Still, the sooner you work out these personal issues, the sooner you will be ready for full-time work. This should bring you income you can count on as well as health insurance and other benefits. Stick with your plan, even when it seems difficult or impossible. Soon you will be on your way to financial independence.

At times, it will take sheer determination, but you can do it. Ask for help when you need it. Find ways to manage your stress. Remind yourself why you have chosen the goals you have. What did you hope to gain? Remembering this may make your effort seem worth while. Always keep the end in sight. Think of all you and your child have to gain.

Major Points

As a teen parent, you may wonder what your future holds. What happens in the future depends how you plan and what preparations you start making now. Looking at your current situation can help you decide where you want the future to take you.

Your first step toward career planning is exploring your career options. What type of work interests you, and what are you looking for in a career? There are many sources of job and career information you can use to help you decide.

Once you have gathered information about a few careers that interest you, it's time to make a decision. Consider your values, skills, and interests when making this choice. Think about job trends and opportunities, too.

Working in your career field is your main long-term career goal. Set subgoals to help you reach this end goal. This will be a step-by-step process. As you reach one goal, move on to the next. Keep doing this until you've planned a path from now until you have a job in your chosen field.

One or more of your career subgoals may involve education and training. First, complete high school, whether by graduating or earning the GED. You might also want to consider school-to-work programs, apprenticeships, occupational training, or college. Get as much education and training as you need to work in your chosen field.

There are also other ways to prepare for your future job. Learn what makes a good employee and develop some of these qualities and skills. A job readiness program could help you do this. Finally, think ahead to barriers you might face. Plan how you'll overcome them. Keep your long-term goal in sight and try to stay motivated.

Chapter 7
Succeeding in
the Workplace

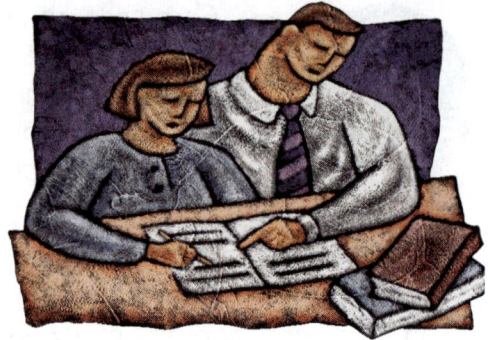

One day, you will be ready to look for your first full-time job. Your job search may take some effort, but don't worry. With patience, planning, and dedication, you will be able to find the right job for you.

This chapter will teach you about some of the tools you can use to secure the job you want. It will also tell you how to succeed on the job once you're hired. As a new employee, you'll want to develop positive work behaviors and learn about your employee rights. Finally, this chapter will suggest ways you can balance the many roles you might have. Achieving this balance will make your life run more smoothly.

Finding the Job You Want

Now you're ready to start looking for a job. It's time to put together the tools you'll need to land the job you want. It may take some searching to find job openings that appeal to you. When you find these, you'll want to sell yourself to your potential employers. It's your job to convince them you would be a good addition to their workplace. Some of the tools you can use to do this are your resume, cover letter, job application, and interview.

The Job Search

When you're ready to look for a job, you may wonder how to begin your search. People find jobs in several ways. Your job search can include some or all of these methods.

Many people get job leads through networking. This means talking with people you know who may be able to steer you toward jobs. See Figure 7-1. It also includes meeting new people who could be potential job contacts. Networking is often the easiest way to open the door to employment.

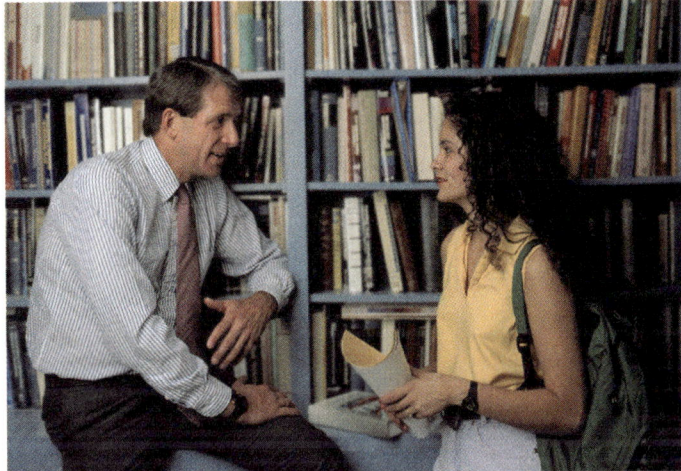

7-1 Asking your teachers if they know of any job leads is an example of networking.

To network, you let people in your network know you are looking for a job. You fill them in on your interests and qualifications. Then you ask if they know of job openings you might pursue. Perhaps your teachers, counselors, or caseworkers can suggest places for you to apply for a job. They may be able to recommend you for specific jobs. They may even be able to put you in touch with employers or help you arrange an interview. You may have a friend who works someplace you'd like to work. Ask if your friend can introduce you to his or her supervisor or help you set up an interview.

Who might you include in your network? This will vary, depending on the people you know. See Figure 7-2. People in your network can help point you in the right direction, recommend you for specific jobs, advise you on your resume, and possibly help you set up interviews. Your network of personal contacts is an excellent place to start your search.

The Internet is another good way to search for work. You can look for Web sites that provide job listings. This is a way to find openings for which you can apply. Some of these sites offer links directly to the companies and agencies with openings. You may be able to submit your resume and apply for the job online.

Who's in Your Network?

Your network includes anyone who might be able to point you toward possible job leads. This might include any of the following people:

* teachers and counselors at your school or training program
* caseworker
* mentors
* parents and their friends and coworkers
* friends
* neighbors
* relatives
* classmates
* former coworkers or employers
* people from your house of worship or other activities

7-2 Your network includes many people, including some you may not have considered before.

You can also use the Internet to help you with other job search tasks. Some Web sites offer advice on resumes, interviews, and career planning. Many companies and agencies have Web sites. You can visit these sites to learn more about the places you want to apply for jobs. This can help you prepare for your interviews.

If you don't have access to the Internet at home, you may be able to go online at your public library, school, or community center. These places often have Internet access and people who can help you find your way online. Once you get started, you'll be amazed at the information available to you online.

Be a little cautious when submitting a resume or any personal information online, however. Make sure the job-search service you're using is a reputable one. Find out what policy the Web site has on protecting the privacy of your personal information. If they have no policy, everyone using the Internet could potentially access this information. Your name, address, telephone number, and Social Security number might no longer be private.

A third job-search method involves reading classified ads. This section of your local newspaper will likely include a list of job openings under the title Help Wanted. In this list, you will find nearby job openings listed by job title. From these ads, you might learn the following:

- ☛ the company hiring and possibly where it's located
- ☛ job title and possibly a description
- ☛ whether the job is full-time or part-time
- ☛ qualifications and experience required
- ☛ salary and benefits information
- ☛ contact information to apply for the job

Also in the classified ads section, you might learn about upcoming job and career fairs. A job fair is an event where employers and job seekers gather to talk about possible job openings. At a job fair, you can talk to many employers about your skills and interests. You can learn about companies and the types of jobs they offer. If you attend a job fair, take plenty of copies of your resume with you. You can give them to employers and maybe even set up some interviews. A job fair is also a good place to network. You can collect the business cards of employers who might become contacts for future job leads.

Finally, you may want to find out if there is a youth services or youth employment center in your area. Youth job centers can be comfortable places to learn about available jobs. If there is a center near you, go there and talk to the counselors. Fill out an application and leave your resume. These types of agencies specialize in helping young people find work. If there's no such center for young people, you might try contacting the local job placement or unemployment office. These offices might have listings of jobs that would interest you.

Evaluating Job Offers

As you start interviewing, think about what you want in a job. This can help you decide which jobs would work best for you. What are your work requirements and preferences? Think about the following questions as you decide:

- ☛ What distance from home can you travel to a job?
- ☛ Do you need full- or part-time work?
- ☛ What hours and days of the week can you work?

☞ What is the minimum level of pay you can accept?

☞ Can you take a job that requires travel or a car?

☞ Can you take a job that requires you to work overtime or be on-call?

Figure 7-3 lists other things to consider as you evaluate job offers and employers. Which of these are most important for you? In some cases, you can be flexible about what you want. For instance, even if you can work on Sundays, you might not prefer to do so. If working Sundays is a requirement of the job you want, you may decide to compromise.

On the other hand, a job may require you to travel a long distance to work. If you have no car or other means of transportation, you will have to turn down the job. Another job may require you to work overtime or be on-call. Unless you can arrange child care that allows you to do this, you will need to refuse the job.

Think through what a job must provide for you and where you are willing to compromise. It is a good idea to have this firmly in mind when you are interviewing.

Before you accept a job, ask for a copy of the employee handbook. Take this home and read it before you take the job. This will help you learn about the employer's policies. The handbook can

What Do I Want in a Job?

Rank these items from most to least important. Number the most important item 1, and so on. Write any other factors you find important in a job, and include these in your ranking.

❑ pleasant coworkers   ❑ good pay   ❑ working with people
❑ pleasant surroundings   ❑ job security   ❑ working independently
❑ opportunity to advance   ❑ flexible hours   ❑ family-friendly policies
❑ desirable location   ❑ employee benefits   ❑ other: _____
❑ variety of tasks   ❑ fair treatment   ❑ other: _____

7-3 Deciding what you want in a job is an important first step.

tell you if the employer is family-friendly. Does the company offer flexible hours or on-site child care? What about other child care assistance? What are the policies on vacation and sick time, as well as maternity leave? The answers to these questions might help you decide whether this is the job for you.

Creating Your Resume

A resume is a document that tells an employer what you have to offer as an employee. In many cases, it will be the first impression you give an employer. Think of it as a sales tool. A strong resume can help get you a job interview. A poorly written one may be tossed out without another glance. For this reason, it's important to take the time to make your resume the best it can be.

You may wonder what your resume should look like. See Figure 7-4 for a sample. Your resume may be set up a little differently from this one, but it will likely have the same basic parts. These are the following:

1. your name, address, and telephone number

2. your job objective— briefly describe the type of work you are seeking

3. education and training you've completed—list all schools attended, areas of study, degrees or certificates earned, and skills you have mastered

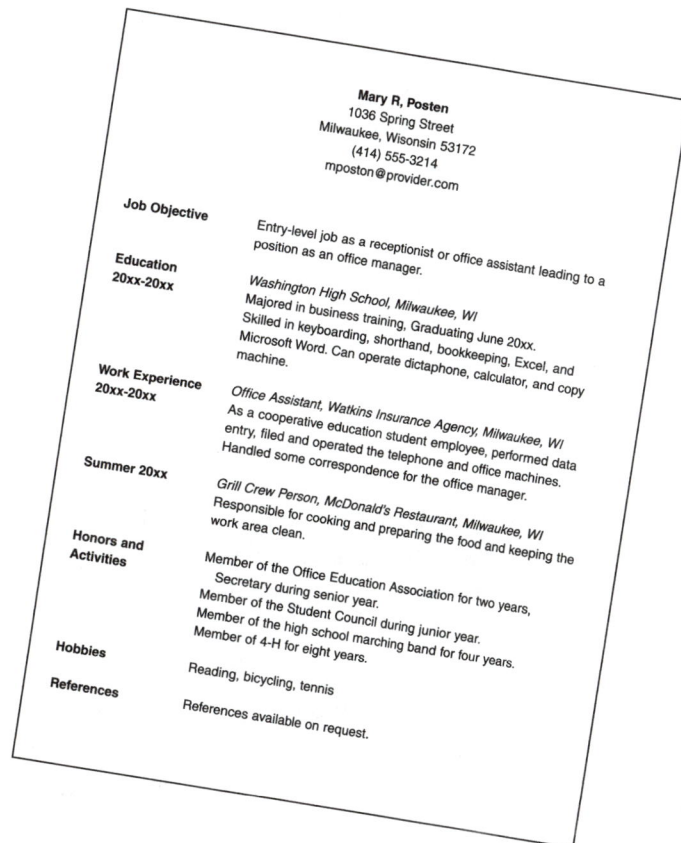

Mary R. Posten
1036 Spring Street
Milwaukee, Wisonsin 53172
(414) 555-3214
mposton@provider.com

Job Objective
Entry-level job as a receptionist or office assistant leading to a position as an office manager.

Education
20xx-20xx
Washington High School, Milwaukee, WI
Majored in business training, Graduating June 20xx.
Skilled in keyboarding, shorthand, bookkeeping, Excel, and Microsoft Word. Can operate dictaphone, calculator, and copy machine.

Work Experience
20xx-20xx
Office Assistant, Watkins Insurance Agency, Milwaukee, WI
As a cooperative education student employee, performed data entry, filed and operated the telephone and office machines. Handled some correspondence for the office manager.

Summer 20xx
Grill Crew Person, McDonald's Restaurant, Milwaukee, WI
Responsible for cooking and preparing the food and keeping the work area clean.

Honors and Activities
Member of the Office Education Association for two years, Secretary during senior year.
Member of the Student Council during junior year.
Member of the high school marching band for four years.
Member of 4-H for eight years.

Hobbies
Reading, bicycling, tennis

References
References available on request.

7-4 A resume should be neat, clean, and error-free. You want your resume to represent you well.

4. previous work experience you've had—list any jobs you've held and describe your responsibilities at each

5. your activities and honors—list volunteer work, activities and programs in which you've participated, honors you've received, scholarships or academic recognition, and good citizen awards

6. your references—on your resume, write the phrase <u>References available upon request</u>

When formatting your resume to send online, don't be fancy. In fact, some formatting, such as lines, fancy fonts, or artwork, may not transmit well. These may make your resume look all jumbled to the employer. This would not make a good impression. Instead, use plain typefaces and a simple layout. This type of resume will transmit the best.

Employers may give less than a minute's attention to each resume, so make sure yours stands out. You can create your resume on a computer. Print it out on high-quality paper. This will give it a professional look. Keep your resume brief and easy-to-read. Use active verbs to describe previous job duties. Look over your final copy closely. Be sure everything lines up and there are no errors. Ask someone else to check your resume, too. Make any needed changes before giving it to a prospective employer. Following these guidelines can help you make the most of this first impression with the employer.

References

A reference is a person who knows you well and is willing to speak on your behalf. Employers want to call your references to learn more about what kind of person you are. This helps them make hiring decisions.

Who will you ask to serve as a reference? Teachers, counselors, or former employers may know you and your work well. Sometimes there are other adults who know your character and qualifications well, too. Never name a relative as your reference. Employers would expect them to be biased in your favor.

Having three references is usually seen as the norm. When you choose people to serve as references for you, be sure to ask their permission. Alert these people when you start a job search. Update them as you gain qualifications and experience. This will allow them to speak knowledgeably about you. It will improve your chances of getting hired.

List your references on a separate sheet from your resume. This sheet should give the name, title, address, and phone number of each person serving as a reference. Give this sheet to employers who ask for it.

Writing a Cover Letter

A cover letter is a letter to a potential employer that is often included with a resume. It is also sometimes called a letter of introduction. This letter lets you tell more than what is contained in your resume. While you can send exactly the same resume to many employers, each cover letter should be unique. It should tell the following:

- how you learned of the position
- why you're interested in the job
- why you're a good match for the job
- description of any enclosures (resume, references, etc.)
- what action you will take or would like to have the employer take to follow up

End the letter by thanking the employer for his or her time in reviewing your letter and resume. See Figure 7-5 for a sample cover letter.

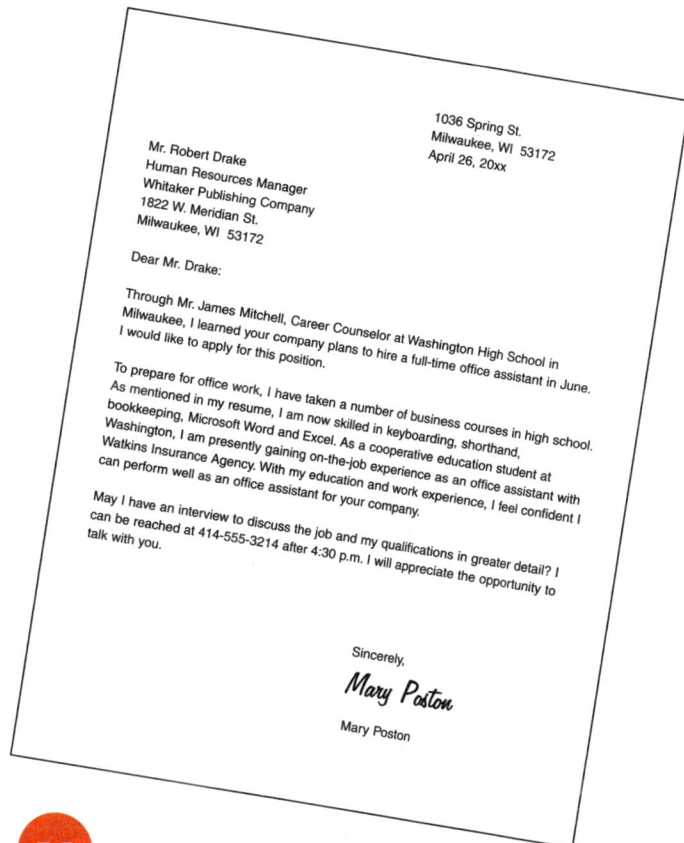

1036 Spring St.
Milwaukee, WI 53172
April 26, 20xx

Mr. Robert Drake
Human Resources Manager
Whitaker Publishing Company
1822 W. Meridian St.
Milwaukee, WI 53172

Dear Mr. Drake:

Through Mr. James Mitchell, Career Counselor at Washington High School in Milwaukee, I learned your company plans to hire a full-time office assistant in June. I would like to apply for this position.

To prepare for office work, I have taken a number of business courses in high school. As mentioned in my resume, I am now skilled in keyboarding, shorthand, bookkeeping, Microsoft Word and Excel. As a cooperative education student at Washington, I am presently gaining on-the-job experience as an office assistant with Watkins Insurance Agency. With my education and work experience, I feel confident I can perform well as an office assistant for your company.

May I have an interview to discuss the job and my qualifications in greater detail? I can be reached at 414-555-3214 after 4:30 p.m. I will appreciate the opportunity to talk with you.

Sincerely,

Mary Poston

Mary Poston

7-5

A cover letter serves as an introduction for your resume. It helps explain why you think you should be considered for the job.

Your letter should sound the way you speak. Use active, interesting words. Be businesslike, yet not stilted or stuffy. Print your cover letter on the same paper you used for your resume. Review the final copy to make sure there are no mistakes. These tips should help you write a cover letter that will make the employer want to read your resume. If you need more help, ask your teacher, counselor, or caseworker for advice.

Completing a Job Application

A prospective employer may ask you to complete a job application. This is a form on which you give potential employers information about yourself. Completing this form means you want to be considered for the job. Employers may base hiring choices in part on how well you fill out the application. Use the job application to make the best impression you can.

There is an art to filling out applications. Practice makes it easier. Study the completed sample in Figure 7-6. Then collect job applications from local businesses. Make copies of these forms so you have plenty to practice with. Fill out each application, using your best handwriting.

When you pick up a job application from an employer, you may be asked to fill it out and turn it in before leaving. To prepare for this possibility, take a blue or black pen with you. Also bring your resume and list of references. You will need this information to complete the form. You may also be asked to leave these for the employer.

If you can take the application with you and bring it back, this may be easier. This way you can make a couple of copies of the form for practice. Fill in the information on the copy and then transfer it to the original. Work slowly so you won't lose your place.

The following are additional tips for completing a job application:

- ☞ Read the entire application before writing on it. Be sure you understand each question before answering. Be careful to write answers in their correct blanks.

☛ Carefully read (and follow) the directions for completing the form.

☛ Complete all the questions on both sides of the form that apply to you.

☛ Write neatly and clearly. Spell correctly.

☛ If you make a mistake, draw a single line through it. Write in the correct answer as neatly as possible as close to the blank as you can.

☛ Be brief and accurate when writing about your education, work history, and past experience.

7-6 A job application provides prospective employers basic information about you and your experience.

☛ Include the names, titles, addresses, and phone numbers of former employers and your references.

Interviewing Well

The next job-seeking tool that can work for you is the interview. This is a meeting between you and a prospective employer to discuss a job opening. It may be your first chance to meet the employer in person. The employer interviews you to learn whether you're the right person for the job.

The interview is an important talk. You may feel nervous about it—this is normal. To put your best foot forward in an interview, you will need to prepare. You can take several steps to be sure you're ready. These include the following:

☞ Before the interview, learn what you can about the employer, company, or organization where you are applying for work. Try to think of ways you would fit into the organization. Be ready to tell what you can contribute.

☞ Think about questions you may be asked. These may include the following: Why are you applying for this job? What qualifies you for the job? What strengths and weaknesses would you bring to the job? What are your career goals? What can you tell me about yourself? Practice answers for these questions ahead of time.

☞ Be familiar with the types of questions a prospective employer cannot ask. These questions are illegal, and you don't have to answer them. See Figure 7-7. Think about how you would respond if you were asked an inappropriate question.

☞ Practice your interviewing techniques with a teacher, friend, or counselor. Try to develop a confident, friendly manner. Try to sound as natural and relaxed as possible.

☞ Prepare a list of questions to ask during the interview. Ask specific questions about the company, job duties, opportunities to advance, and employee policies. Avoid asking about salary and benefits too early in the interview. This makes it seem you're more interested in the money than in the job or the company. The interviewer might tell you about these topics, or you can ask when you're offered the job.

☞ If you're not familiar with the interview location, ask the employer for directions. If you will go to the interview by car, ask where to park and what the fee is. If you will take public transportation, check the schedule ahead of time. Either way, make a practice trip at the same time of day as the interview. This gives you an idea how long the trip will be. Allow even more time than this on the day of the interview— you don't want to cut it too close.

☞ Gather the materials you will need to take with you to the interview. These may include a pen, your resume, a completed job application, your transcript from high school or college, a list of references, and your Social Security card. Also bring your list of questions to ask. You may want to place these items carefully in a folder or envelope so they will stay neat.

Questions Employers Cannot Ask

It is illegal for a prospective employer to ask you any of the following questions. Think ahead of time about how you will respond if you are asked these questions.

* Can you attach a current photograph of yourself to your application?
* What is your skin, hair, or eye color?
* What is your race?
* What nationality are you, your spouse, or your parents?
* What is your ancestry?
* What language do you and your family speak at home?
* What is your native language?
* Where were you born?
* Where were your parents or relatives born?
* Are you a naturalized citizen?
* Do you have any children?
* What child care arrangements do you have?
* Do you plan to have children?
* Are you single, married, divorced, or widowed?
* Would you rather be addressed as Miss, Ms., or Mrs.?
* What is your religion?
* What church do you attend?
* What religious holidays do you observe?
* What is your age?
* When were you born?
* Do you have any disabilities?
* To what organizations or clubs do you belong?

7-7 If you are asked one of these questions during an interview, what would you do?

On the Day of the Interview

Preparing for the interview will help the day go smoothly. There are many points to keep in mind about the interview day, however.

First, look to your appearance and the impression you make. Wear clean, pressed clothes that are appropriate for an interview. Be sure your hair is clean and well groomed. You can wear some makeup, but don't apply it too heavily.

Don't take anyone with you. This would not be appropriate, and the employer would likely count it against you. Arrange ahead of time to have someone care for your child. If someone will be driving you to the interview, ask this person to wait for you outside the building.

Arrive five to ten minutes early. Tell the receptionist who you are and whom you have an appointment to see. Wait patiently until the interviewer asks for you. Try to relax. Greet the interviewer with a firm handshake and a smile. Make eye contact with him or her.

When answering the interviewer's questions, take your time. If you'd like a minute to think about your answer, say so. Don't dawdle, but don't rush, either.

When the interview ends, thank the interviewer for his or her time. Be sure he or she knows where and how to contact you. In a few cases, you will be offered the job at the end of the interview. If this happens, ask for a day or two to think it over unless you are absolutely sure you want the job.

Most times, you will hear about the job later. The interviewer may have other interviews scheduled or want to think over your qualifications. If he or she doesn't mention when the decision will be made, you can ask.

Within a day or two after the interview, write a thank-you letter to the interviewer. This should be short and to the point. Tell the employer you enjoyed the chance to learn about the company and talk with him or her about the job. Express your interest in the job and mention you look forward to hearing from the employer soon.

If you do not hear within two or three weeks, you may want to follow up with a phone call. This would be appropriate unless you have been asked not to call.

Achieving Job Success

Starting a new job is a major life change. With this new responsibility, many other things in your life will change, too. It will take time to adjust to the changes your new job will bring. Your child and your family will have to adjust, too. Being patient with one another can make this transition a little smoother. See Figure 7-8.

When you start your new job, you may feel overwhelmed by all the changes. Stick with your job and give it a fair chance. You will adjust in a shorter time than you think. Keep in mind working is your road to supporting yourself and becoming independent.

Learning your job and getting used to your new schedule may take some time. Finding time to meet the demands of home and family will be a challenge. You'll have less time to do homemaking and parenting tasks than you did before. If your family, partner, or friends can help with some of these tasks, it will ease the load.

7-8 When you first start working, try to spend what time you can just enjoying your child.

Finding child care will be a top priority. Many teen parents choose relatives, child care centers, or family child care homes to care for their children while they work. When you feel comfortable about your child's care, you can focus better on your new job. (See another title in this series, Helping Your Child Grow and Develop, to learn more about choosing child care.)

Developing Positive Work Behaviors

If this new job is your first, you may feel unsure what kind of behavior is required on a job. Ask a trusted adult, teacher,

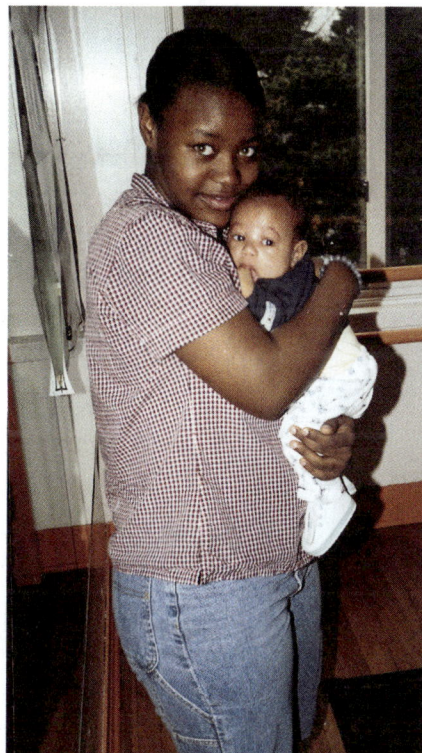

counselor, or caseworker for advice. Coworkers can often help you, too. Their insight may help you develop work behaviors that will lead to success on the job.

You are likely to keep your job and get promoted if you do the following:

- ☛ Arrive every workday early or at least on time. If you must be late or miss work, call your employer as soon as you're aware of this. Good employees miss work only rarely and for very good reasons. If you want to take vacation days or time without pay, ask permission beforehand. Be as flexible as possible.
- ☛ Come to work clean, neat, and dressed for the job. Clothes need to fit well and be appropriate for the workplace.
- ☛ Accept responsibility and do your very best on the job. Find out what is expected of you and deliver.
- ☛ Show enthusiasm for your job. Let your employer know you're grateful to have a job and pleased to work for him or her. Show an interest in succeeding and advancing on the job.
- ☛ Make it a point to get along well with your supervisor, coworkers, and customers or clients. If you need improvement in this area, ask your supervisor to help you.
- ☛ Follow orders and directions willingly. If the directions aren't clear, ask your supervisor to explain further. If you run into a problem, ask for help right away.
- ☛ Keep busy and stay on task. Ask for extra work when you have free time. Avoid looking bored or watching the clock. Work until quitting time. Don't put away your things or leave early.

As well as behaviors you should develop, there are some you should avoid. These will lead to trouble on the job and perhaps even get you fired. See Figure 7-9.

Your new job may have a probationary period. During this time, you will be evaluated on the work you do and how well you fit into the workplace. Ask questions and request any help you need. At the end of this period, your employer will decide whether to keep you on in your present position. This is most likely if you do your job well and have a good attitude.

Work Behaviors to Avoid

You're likely to lose your job if you do one or more of the following:

* miss work frequently
* usually come to work late
* often appear tired, disinterested, or bored
* permit friends to come by or call you at work
* use drugs or alcohol before work or on the job
* lose your temper with bosses, coworkers, or customers
* let personal issues and problems interfere with your work
* use foul or abusive language at work
* argue with supervisors, coworkers, or customers
* fail to serve customers or clients well
* act rude, disrespectful, or disruptive

7-9 Using these behaviors in the workplace can lead you to be fired quickly.

Even after the probationary period, you will be evaluated from time to time. Many employees have annual (once yearly) evaluations. For others, this may happen more often. It is a time when your supervisor can share with you what he or she thinks of your work. You will be rated in areas such as productivity (how much work you do), job knowledge, initiative (how willing you are to take on extra tasks), and attitude. High scores on your evaluation may earn you a raise or promotion. Less-high scores point out areas where you need to improve. Very low scores can be cause for dismissal.

Your supervisor has the right to tell you what to do on the job. This person will give you directions, make suggestions, and correct your mistakes. He or she may or may not be nice about this. If you have a difficult boss, remember self-control. Be as professional as you can. Treat your supervisor with respect and courtesy at all times. This is true even when he or she gives you directions you don't like or corrects you in front of others.

Resist the urge to tell your supervisor off. This is not tolerated in the workplace and can cause you to lose your job. Instead, find a respectful way to express your negative feelings to your boss. If you find it hard to control your temper, remember what is at stake. Choose a wiser, more responsible approach.

When Your Job Isn't Working Out

When you're first hired, you and your employer have the best of hopes. Both of you hope you will be well suited for the job and the organization. You hope you'll be able to learn the job quickly and do it well. You hope you'll be satisfied with the job and enjoy it. Often, this is the case. Unfortunately, sometimes it is not.

If you begin to feel unhappy in your job, take this as a warning sign. Try to determine what about the job is not meeting your expectations. Brainstorm ways you could improve the situation or your attitude. Try these ideas. If they don't solve the problem, you may want to talk to your supervisor. Maybe the two of you can figure out a way to make things better. Give his or her suggestions a try. Try to stick with your job at least six months. Sometimes it takes this long to fully adjust and learn your duties. Your negative feelings may ease in time.

If all else fails, it may be time to look for another job. You will be happier when you find work that fits you better. It is important to handle this situation in the most businesslike way you can. You do not want to build a poor reputation. You may need your current supervisor to serve as a reference. Keep on the best terms with this person as you can. Do not do anything that will get you fired. Avoid quitting your job until you have found another job. Once you find a new job, treat your previous employer with courtesy and respect. Give at least two weeks' notice of your plans to leave. End the job on the best terms possible.

Knowing Your Employee Rights

As an employee, you have certain legal rights. These rights are protected by law. Your employer may also have other policies that give you rights. Know what your rights are so you can protect yourself. Find out what to do if you feel these rights are being violated.

When you start a new job, ask for a copy of the employee handbook. The handbook should outline policies and practices that apply to all employees. It will also explain the terms of the benefits you are entitled to receive. You have the right to fair treatment as described in the handbook. If there is no handbook, ask for an explanation of company policies the employer follows. This will let you know what to expect.

Suppose a supervisor doesn't observe your rights according to the stated policies. Discuss the matter with someone higher in the company, if you can. Union members can usually submit their cases to the union grievance committee. If a company seriously ignores your legal rights, this can be grounds for a lawsuit. However, suing should only come as a last resort for serious violations. See Figure 7-10 for a summary of laws that protect you in the workplace.

Laws That Protect You in the Workplace

Law	Key Provisions
Civil Rights Act of 1964	❖ bans employment discrimination based on race, color, religion, sex, or national origin. ❖ prohibits sexual harassment in the workplace.
Civil Rights Act of 1991	❖ strengthens the ban on employment discrimination based on race, color, religion, sex, or national origin. ❖ provids greater damage awards for workers who successfully sue employers because of discrimination or sexual harassment. ❖ expands the definition of job-related discrimination and sexual harassment.
Americans with Disabilities Act of 1990	❖ prohibits employment discrimination on the basis of disabilities that do not interfere with job performance. ❖ requires employers to make reasonable space and access accommodations for disabled workers.
Equal Pay Act of 1963	❖ prohibits pay discrimination on the basis of gender. ❖ requires men and women to receive the same rate of pay for work that needs equal skill, effort, and responsibility and is performed under similar working conditions.
Fair Labor Standards Act of 1938	❖ sets the rate and rules regarding the minimum wage and overtime pay. (Several amendments to this law have been passed to adjust the rate and rules.) ❖ establishes regulations regarding work by minors (people under age 18).

(Continued)

7-10 This summary of employment legislation outlines some of the protections you have as an employee.

Laws That Protect You in the Workplace

Law	Key Provisions
Family and Medical Leave Act of 1993	❖ requires most employers to allow up to 12 weeks unpaid leave each year for the birth or adoption of a child, to care for a close relative with a serious health condition, or to recover from the employee's own serious health condition. ❖ requires employers to restore returning employees to their jobs or to jobs with equal status, benefits, and pay.
Federal Unemployment Tax Act	❖ requires employers to pay unemployment tax on wages to employees who work more than 20 weeks or who receive $1,500 or more in wages in any given quarter.
Health Insurance Portability and Accountability Act	❖ limits the loss of insurance coverage for employees who leave one job for another. ❖ eliminates waiting periods for preexisting conditions when employees change jobs.
Consolidated Omnibus Budget Reconciliation Act (COBRA)	❖ provides for the continuation of group health insurance for employees who leave a job. Employee can be covered at the group rate for up to 18 months, but must pay the premium and up to 2% more for administrative costs.
Consumer Credit Protection Act	❖ limits the amount of an employee's wages that can be garnished. ❖ prohibits employers from firing an employee for wage garnishments for any one debt.
Employee Retirement Income Security Act (ERISA)	❖ sets standards and requirements for certain fringe benefits and employee-sponsored pension and retirement plans. ❖ requires employers to give employees descriptive materials, benefits information, and annual reports about their companies.
Occupational Safety and Health Act (OSHA)	❖ requires employers to meet federal and/or state requirements involving safety in the workplace.
Workers Adjustment and Retraining Notification Act	❖ requires employers with 100 or more full-time workers to give employees 60 days advance notice of plant closings or mass layoffs.
Workers' Compensation Benefits	❖ requires employers to pay worker's compensation insurance. ❖ grants workers the right to specific benefits if injured and/or disabled on the job. Benefits may include payment of medical expenses, income, and permanent disability settlements. These vary from state to state.

7-10   *Continued*

Employment-at-will is one work arrangement that gives only limited employee rights. In this arrangement, either party can end the job at any time without a reason. An employer could fire you (or you could quit) without giving notice or a reason. This arrangement offers little job security. It is most common in entry-level or temporary jobs. As you move up in the workplace, you're likely to find a job with more security.

Even employees-at-will have some protection against wrongful firing, though. Limitations on an employer's right to fire vary from state to state. You may want to find out your state's laws regarding this. Any of the following reasons might be a wrongful firing:

- ☛ you recently filed a claim for workers' compensation benefits
- ☛ you've been ordered by the court to serve on a jury
- ☛ you refuse the sexual advances of a coworker or superior
- ☛ you receive a garnishment or wage-withholding order for child support payments
- ☛ you refuse to commit perjury when requested by your employer to do so
- ☛ you report an employer's illegal acts to the authorities
- ☛ you file criminal charges against a coworker for acts committed in the course of employment

Firing an employee based on race, color, religion, gender, national origin, age, or disability is also illegal. In cases of wrongful firing, employers can be sued. If you think you may have a wrongful firing case, seek legal advice.

Knowing your legal rights help protect you from an employer's wrongful actions. If your rights are violated in the workplace, don't suffer in silence. Speak up so the matter can be corrected.

Balancing Your Many Roles

Your success in the workplace depends in part on your ability to find balance in your life. There are many roles you must fill. Each of these brings with it certain responsibilities. At times you may feel overwhelmed with all you have to do and be. This is normal. What matters most is how you respond to this feeling.

Ideally, you will find a way to relax and think of ways to make things fit together more smoothly. You'll plan ways to fit everything in as best you can. At times, though, this can be difficult. You may be more focused on the stress you feel than on finding a solution. In these times, you may have to remind yourself to slow down for a minute to regroup.

It is not easy to take care of a child, study, work, and do housework. You also must find time for yourself as well as for your baby, family, partner, and friends. With all these roles, there is quite a demand for your limited time. That is why it's important to manage your time well.

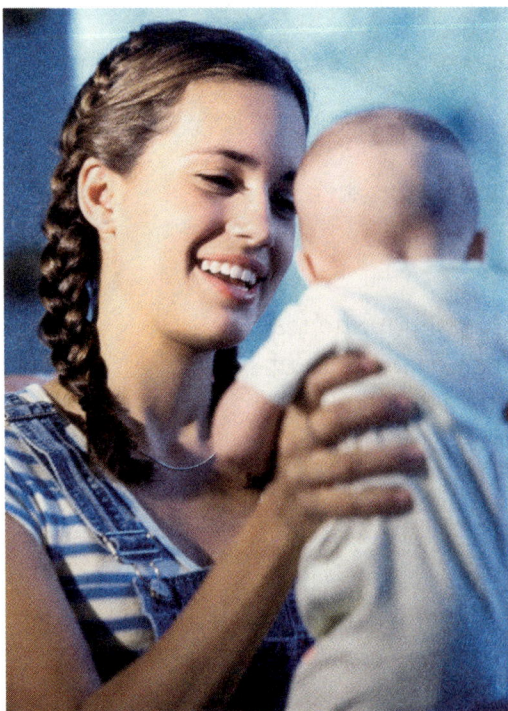

Looking at all your roles with a "big picture" view may add to your tension. Imagine listing everything you have to do in every aspect of your life. Even thinking about such a massive list can cause stress! It may be easier to think of each role separately first. This breaks your tasks into smaller pieces you can manage. Consider what is needed from you in each area before making a big-picture plan.

In most everything you do, you will have your child in mind. You are a parent—this must take top priority. Your child depends on you to provide care and supervision for him. See Figure 7-11. He needs you to teach, guide, and discipline him. Maybe most of all, he needs you to love him and spend time with him. All these tasks take time and energy.

7-11 Your parenting role is one of the most important and rewarding roles you will have in life.

If you work or are in school, you'll be away from your young child much of the day. This can be hard for both of you. At first it may be tough to manage your feelings. If you're like many mothers, you will think of your child throughout the day. He'll miss you, too. If he cries when you leave him at child care, it can be hard to remember why you're doing all this. You may feel guilty. Keep in mind you're doing your best to give him a good life. The work you're doing will help you provide for him. Your schooling will pave the way for a future job that will support him.

One way to handle these feelings is to make the most of the time you have together. Set aside some time every day just to be with your child. Make it a time for fun and connection. You may only be able to spare half an hour each day or a couple hours during the week. These times will be special for both of you. Try to build this time into your routine so the two of you can count on it. In your special time, you may want to read stories, cuddle, listen to music, or just be close. As your child grows, these times can be a chance to talk about the day's events. This will be a good way to know what's going on in your child's life. It will help you stay connected.

School brings with it a different set of responsibilities. It will be essential for you to attend classes regularly. Missing class will only cause you to fall behind. It will be harder to do well if you're often absent. For this reason, reliable child care is a must. It's also good to have a workable backup plan for child care.

Along with attending classes, you'll need to set aside time for study. Some moms choose to study after putting their children to bed. As your child gets older, you might be able to do your homework when he does his. This depends on how much of your help he needs with his studies. One thing is certain—you'll need to stay up-to-date on school assignments. If you start to let your homework slide, you'll soon find yourself unable to catch up.

You can ease the stress of school by treating it as a job. See Figure 7-12. Stay organized. Take good notes. Pay attention in class. Study for tests a little each day rather than cramming. Begin work on long-term projects early—don't wait until the last minute. Keep your teachers informed if you must miss class or

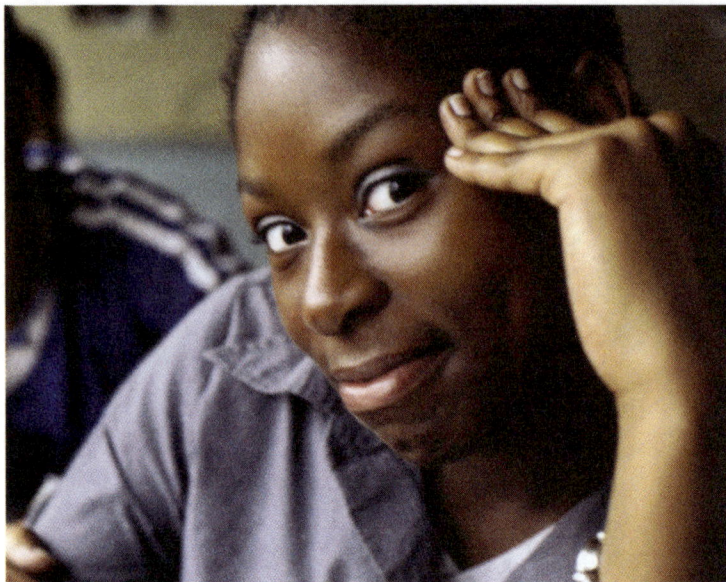

7-12 Paying attention in class makes school much easier and decreases your stress level.

are having trouble keeping up with your work. These tips will help you stay on track in school.

Work may be another of your big responsibilities. You may be working at a full- or part-time job now. Whether you're married or single, being a working mom is a challenge. Thousands of parents before you have done it, though, and you can do it, too. Women with children under six years old make up more than half of the workforce. In fact, most mothers work outside the home at some point. This is especially true for single moms.

If you work, a large chunk of your day will go to your job. First, you will spend time getting ready for work. Next, you may have to travel to child care and then on to work. Be sure to plan enough time for these activities, because getting to work on time each day is vital. During work hours, your employer expects you to give your job the attention it deserves. This, too, takes energy. Some days, you may feel drained by the time you leave work. Of course, you'll still have to travel to pick up your child and get home.

Work is often the area in which parents have the least amount of flexibility. For the most part, you'll have to plan everything else around your job. If your employer has family-friendly policies, this may not be as big a problem for you. You might be able to set your own hours or do some of your work from home. This would make it much easier to balance your work and other roles.

Personal time is also important. Since you became a parent, this may be the one area that has changed the most dramatically. Even though you have a child to care for, you need time alone, too. When trying to fit in extra activities and tasks, many parents cut their personal time first. Actually, having personal time renews your energy.

Be sure to take the time to eat well, rest enough, and be physically active. Seek the medical care you need. When you're in good health, you will have more energy and patience to deal with the world. Being run down will only make things harder for you. Taking care of yourself is not selfish. In fact, it allows you to take better care of other people and responsibilities.

Set aside time for yourself, even if it's just minutes each day or a few hours each week. Ask someone to watch your child for a couple hours. If no one can help, go in the other room for a while when your child is asleep. Don't feel bad about taking the time you need. This helps you be a better mother. It relieves stress so you don't take it out on your child. Use this time to recharge yourself by doing something you enjoy. It may be as simple as taking a long bath, going for a walk, or reading a book. See Figure 7-13.

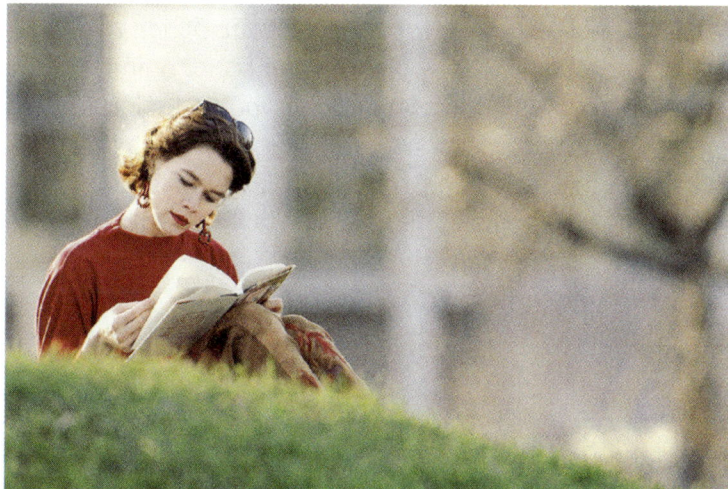

7-13 Taking care of your other responsibilities will be easier if you remember to devote some personal time to yourself once in a while.

Your relationships with others are important, too. You may be close to your family, partner, and friends. Relationships can be a great source of support. Sharing your concerns with others can make them seem easier to handle. Having people you can ask for help can give you a sense of security. Relationships also take time and effort, though. Giving this attention and energy can be hard if you feel overwhelmed with other tasks. You might feel guilty about taking time for fun when you have so much to do.

It can be refreshing to plan special time with your friends or partner. You may really enjoy their company. For a while, it may take your mind off all you have to do. This can reduce stress. You won't want to ignore your other responsibilities, though. One way to compromise is to plan some get-togethers that include both your friends and your child. This can be especially fun if some of your friends are parents, too. They can bring their children to play with your child. This gives you a social life and lets you be with your child at the same time.

Balance is the key. Don't let your relationships take too much time or focus from your other tasks. In a healthy relationship, each person respects the other's limits. There will be giving and taking on both sides. Choose your relationships carefully. People who truly care about you have your best interest at heart. They won't do anything to jeopardize your success, but you'll have to voice your limits. This means saying no to an invitation if you still have homework to do.

Maintaining your home is one final piece to fit into your busy life. Even if you live with your partner or parents, you'll probably have some chores to do. Keeping a house in order takes a lot of time, but there are ways to make it easier. Decide how you want to handle tasks such as budgeting, paying bills, laundry, ironing, shopping, cooking, and cleaning. Some people do a little each day. Others put aside a block of time each week for these chores. Try both ways and then do what works best for you.

Putting It All Together

Think of your roles as pieces of a puzzle. Your goal is to take these separate pieces and arrange them in a way that gives you a good fit. Solving this puzzle is a trial-and-error process. You may need to adjust in one area to improve in another.

The 24 hours you're given each day may not seem like enough time for all there is to do. That's because they're not. Your first step in balancing your roles is to realize you're not perfect. Accept that it is not possible for you to do everything in all areas of your life each day. You will have to juggle your various roles. Some days the housework may have to slide. Another day your homework may not get done. On a third day, you may not have time for yourself or friends. This is normal. You can still have a healthy and successful life if you keep balance in mind.

You will need to prioritize. This means you set priorities, or rank things in order of their importance to you. Your top priorities are those that matter most. When faced with a time crunch, decide what you care about most and let the rest go. Let your priorities be your guide as you try to manage your limited time.

Support is also essential. Call on family members to help you. You may have parents, grandparents, siblings, aunts, uncles, and cousins who can assist. For many young moms, family is the best source of support. Often, they can provide emotional, practical, and financial support. Your family can't help if you don't let them know what you need, though. Be sure to ask for what you need.

If your family isn't supportive, you may be able to build a circle of close friends and coworkers who will offer their support. In time, these people may seem like family to you. Get to know other young parents. Talking with them can relieve stress. These friends may share many of your concerns or be able to offer ideas about what has worked well for them.

Find a support group for young moms. This could be a formal support group or just a few people who choose to get together and talk. In this group, you can share your thoughts and experiences with others who can relate. Knowing others face some of the same challenges you do can lift your spirits. If there are no support groups in your area, consider starting one. This could help both you and others in your area who share your concerns.

You can also use the Internet to find information and support. Go online and look up <u>single mothers</u>, <u>teen parents</u>, or <u>working mothers</u> on a search engine. You should come up with quite a few Web sites you can access. This should be a good source of up-to-date information for you.

Another key to balancing your life is using your time wisely. By improving your time-management skills, you may be able to fit in more activities you want to do. You may also feel less overwhelmed if you budget your time. See Figure 7-14 for tips you can use.

It's also important to manage the stress you feel. Often it helps to identify your stressors and high-stress times. When do you feel stressed? What triggers you to feel this way? Once you're aware of your stressors, you can plan to avoid or minimize them. Preparing for a stressful event such as an exam or job interview can also make a difference. Also think about what time of day

Managing Your Time

As a young parent, you will have to make good use of your time to meet all your responsibilities. The following tips can help you manage time well:

❖ Organize your space. Find a place for the things you need to do such as studying. Reorganize closets, cupboards, and drawers to help you find the things you need. This saves time, which can help reduce stress.

❖ Use a calendar to help you keep track of appointments and special events. Pick a large wall calendar with enough space to write all the things you must do and remember. This will help you plan and organize your time.

❖ Establish routines for bedtimes, mornings, weekends, holidays, and other times that can be hectic. Most children thrive on a routine. They like to know what to expect.

❖ Keep close track of your time. Over a period of a few days, record how you spend all your time throughout the day. Review your records to see areas in which you waste time. Form a plan for using this time more wisely.

❖ Create a time budget. Set specific times to be with your child. Make enough time for study or job-related activities. Plan for the hours needed for household chores, too. Try to schedule time for yourself into your day. Include activities with friends or your partner if you can. Writing out your plan may help you fit in all that matters to you.

❖ Record your life plans and goals on paper. List your personal, parental, financial, and career goals. Outline the steps you must take to achieve each one. Review your goals often. Use them to motivate you when times seem rough.

7-14 Using your time wisely can help you get more accomplished in the limited time you have.

you're most likely to feel stress. For some it is the supper hour. Others find more stress in the morning rush. Plan ways to make this high-stress time easier.

As you step into the work world, you have much to do and consider. The future is full of possibility, but it depends on what you do to make it work for you. It will not always be easy, but you can manage your life. You can prepare to provide for yourself and your child. You've already developed some of the tools you need. Continue to master other new skills. The life you're living also sets an example for your child. Have courage as you rise to the challenges of being a young parent. You can do it.

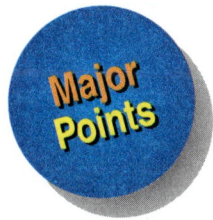

Major Points

☛ Searching for a job may take some time and energy. There are many ways you can conduct your job search. These include networking, using the Internet, reading the classified ads, and visiting job search services and employment offices.

☛ When you find a job opening for which you want to apply, it's your job to convince the employer you would be a good addition to the workplace. Some of the tools you can use to do this are your resume, cover letter, job application, and interview.

☛ Being hired is an exciting achievement. It's the first step to job success. Starting a job requires some adjustments, though. In time, you will learn your new job and get used to your new schedule. Until then, try to be patient with yourself and others around you.

☛ To become a successful and valued employee, you'll need to develop positive work behaviors. You'll want to meet or exceed the employer's expectations about the job you can do and the positive manner in which you can do it. This may take practice, but it will be well worth it in the long run.

☛ As a worker, you have certain rights that are protected by law. Other rights are granted to you through the employer's company policies. Know what these rights are so you can be sure you're being treated fairly and appropriately. If your rights are being violated, speak up and take action to solve the problem.

☛ One final key to job success and happiness is finding balance in your life. Much is expected of you, but you can keep all these demands in perspective. By working to fit your responsibilities together, you can reduce stress and find harmony in your life.

Glossary

A

abortion. Removing an embryo or fetus from the uterus to end a pregnancy. (2)

abstinence. A decision to postpone entering a sexual relationship. (2)

adoption. Legal process through which birthparents transfer their role as parents to adoptive parents. (2)

adoptive parents. People who take on the parenting role as a result of the adoption process. (2)

advertisement. A message paid for by a company to promote goods or services it wants to sell; also called an ad. (4)

Aid to Families with Dependent Children (AFDC) program. Former federal aid program that was replaced by the Temporary Assistance to Needy Families (TANF) program. (1)

annual percentage rate (APR). The actual rate of interest charged for credit figured on a yearly basis. (5)

annulment. Court order that dissolves a marriage as though it never existed based on an approved reason. (2)

apprenticeship. A combination of on-the-job training and classroom learning that teaches people the highly specialized skills they will need to work in the craft or trade industries. (6)

associate degree. Type of degree offered by a community college or junior college; usually earned in two years. (6)

ATM card. Card used to make financial transactions at an ATM machine. (5)

automated teller machine (ATM). Machine that allows you to use a card to electronically deposit or withdraw money from your account. (5)

automobile insurance. Various types of insurance coverage that protect you from the financial risks of owning a car. (5)

B

bachelor's degree. Type of degree offered by a four-year college or university. (6)

beneficiaries. People named in a life insurance policy to collect benefits if the insured person dies. (5)

birthparents. The parents to whom a child is born. (2)

blank endorsement. Type of endorsement that includes only your signature and perhaps your account number. (5)

browser. Tool that helps guide a person through Web sites. (1)

budget. A written plan that allows you to manage spending and reach financial goals. (3)

C

cash advance. Name given to money borrowed in a credit card loan. (5)

cash credit. Type of credit that is given in a loan from a creditor. (5)

cash value policy. Type of life insurance policy that builds cash value over the life of the policy as well as paying benefits at death. (5)

checkbook register. Small booklet in which you record all transactions involving your checking account and keep track of the account balance. (5)

check card. Another name for a debit card. (5)

check credit loan. Cash credit loan in which you use a check to borrow money from a creditor. (5)

checking account. Bank account that lets you deposit money and then write checks on the account. (5)

child abuse. Intentional injury or pattern of injuries to a child; can be physical, emotional, or sexual. (2)

child custody. Rights that can be given by the court to parents who live apart regarding their child. (2)

child neglect. Failure to meet a child's basic physical and emotional needs. (2)

Child Support Enforcement (CSE) Office. Government office that was formed to help residential parents locate absent parents and establish paternity; this office also helps these parents obtain and enforce the collection of child support payments. (2)

child support payments. Court-ordered payments made by a nonresidential parent to the residential parent for the support of the children they have together. (2)

collateral. An item of value you own and pledge to the creditor to secure a loan. (5)

commercial. Name for an advertisement that is broadcast on TV or radio. (4)

common law marriage. Type of marriage created when a couple lives together and presents themselves in public as husband and wife; not legal in all states. (2)

community resources. Resources you earn access to by being a member of your town or city. (3)

consent form. The legal document that makes an adoption final; must be signed by the birthparents. (2)

cosigner. A person with a strong credit rating who signs a loan contract with you, promising to repay if you don't repay as agreed. (5)

coverage. Another name for insurance protection. (5)

covered losses. Losses that are included in your insurance policy and would be paid for by the insurance company. (5)

cover letter. A letter you write to a potential employer that is often included with a resume. (7)

credit. An agreement with a creditor that lets you buy or borrow now and pay later. (5)

credit card loan. Cash credit loan in which you use a credit card to borrow money from a creditor. (5)

creditors. People and companies to whom you owe money; companies that grant you credit. (3)

credit rating. The summary of your financial history that is available to potential creditors; your financial reputation. (5)

custodial parent. Parent with whom a child resides; residential parent. (2)

D

debit card. Card you can use to buy goods or services using money from your account and use as an ATM card; also called a check card. (5)

deductible. The part of your losses you must pay before you can collect anything from the insurance company. (5)

deposit. To put money into your checking or savings account. (5)

determination. Committing to hold firmly to the plan you've chosen; a human resource. (3)

Dietary Guidelines for Americans. A set of suggestions for healthful eating created by the U.S. Department of Agriculture (USDA) and the U.S. Department of Health and Human Services. (4)

divorce. Formal end of a marriage as declared by the court. (2)

domestic violence. Physical, emotional, or sexual harm a person does to someone close to him or her. (2)

down payment. Amount paid to a creditor in advance to secure the loan. (5)

E

Earned Income Tax Credit. A tax credit offered by the IRS to low-income taxpayers to supplement their wages. (6)

emancipation. Court action that grants a teen most of the legal rights of adult. (2)

employment-at-will. Work arrangement that offers only limited employee rights. (7)

endorse. To sign your name on the back of a check, and in some cases, give your account number and directions to the bank about how to handle the check. (5)

exclusions. Losses that are not covered and would not be paid by your insurance policy. (5)

executor. The person named by the writer of the will to carry out the terms of that will after the writer's death. (2)

expenses. All the amounts of money you must pay. (3)

F

fault divorce. Type of divorce in which one or both partners must prove grounds in order for the court to grant the divorce. (2)

final adoption hearing. The court hearing at which an adoption is declared complete and final. (2)

final decree of adoption. Court-issued document that states an adoption is legal and final. (2)

finance charges. Interest and any other amounts charged by the creditor as part of the credit agreement. (5)

fixed expense. An expense that comes due at a set time (and often a set amount) each month or year. (3)

flexible expense. An expense that offers some leeway about when you can pay for it. (3)

flexibility. Being ready and able to adapt to change; a human resource. (3)

full warranty. Type of warranty that provides the most protection in case of product failure. (4)

G

garnishment. Court order that can be sent to a person's employer and requires the employer to withhold part of the employee's wages and send them to the court; often done with child support payments. (2)

General Educational Development (GED) program. Federal education program through which a person can take an exam to earn a general equivalency diploma (GED). (1)

general equivalency diploma (GED). Diploma earned by passing the General Educational Development (GED) exam; seen by many as equal to a high school diploma. (1)

generic products. Type of product that is sold in a plain package without a brand name; offered at lower prices than store brands or national brands. (4)

goal. A statement of what you want to accomplish. (3)

graduate degree. Advanced degree that requires study beyond the bachelor's degree. (6)

grant. Federal, state, or local money that is given to low-income students to help them pay for college. (6)

guardian. Person appointed by the court to assume legal parenting responsibilities for a child if the parents die intestate. (2)

H

health insurance. Type of insurance that helps you pay for the medical care you need to be healthy. (5)

homeowner's insurance. Type of insurance that protect your home and possessions against the risks listed in the policy. (5)

human resources. Tools that come from within yourself or another person that can help you reach your goals. (3)

I

immediate goals. Goals that must be met right away, within a few days or weeks. (3)

impulse buys. Purchases made on the spur of the moment with little thought. (4)

informal adoption. Arrangement in which a parent sends a child to live with a relative, either temporarily or permanently; not recognized by law as an adoption. (2)

installment account. Sales credit account that lets you buy a costly item and pay for it over time. (5)

installment loan. Cash credit loan that lets you repay in regular monthly payments. (5)

insurance. An agreement you make to pay an insurance company in return for their promise to share with you the risks of a covered financial loss. (5)

insurance policy. Your contract with an insurance company regarding your coverage. (5)

interest. Fee you pay a creditor for the use of loaned money. (5)

interest income. Interest you earn; paid to you by the bank for keeping your money on deposit. (5)

internship. A short-term work and learning experience in a particular career field. (6)

interview. A meeting between you and a prospective employer to discuss a job opening. (7)

intestate. Term used when a person dies without having written a will. (2)

issuer. Bank, post office, or business that sells money orders. (5)

J

job application. A form on which you give a potential employer information about yourself. (7)

job fair. An event in which employers and job seekers gather to talk about possible job opportunities. (7)

job readiness program. A program that helps people take the beginning steps toward full-time work. (6)

joint custody. Custody arrangement in which both parents share legal and/or physical custody of the children. (2)

L

legal custody. The right of a parent to make decisions about his or her child's welfare. (2)

legally binding. Describes an agreement that can be upheld in court if needed. (2)

legal separation. Court-approved agreement made by spouses to live apart. (2)

life insurance. Type of insurance coverage that protects your family against the loss of income they would experience if you died. (5)

limited warranty. Type of warranty that offers some protection against product failure but is less complete than a full warranty. (4)

long-term goals. Goals that take more than a year to reach. (3)

M

management. The process of making wise use of what you have to meet your needs and wants. (3)

marketplace. Term used to describe the group of all sellers of goods and services worldwide. (4)

material resources. All the money and objects you own or can use to help reach your goals. (3)

Medicaid program. Federal aid program that pays health care costs for needy individuals and families. (1)

mentor. In a school-to-work program, a person from the worksite assigned to guide the student. (6)

mid-term goal. A goal that takes anywhere from several months to a year to complete. (3)

minimum payment. The lowest amount the creditor will allow you to pay on your credit account for a particular statement period. (5)

minimum wage. The lowest hourly wage employers are allowed to pay. (6)

money order. Piece of paper on which the issuer orders that a specific amount of money be paid to the payee. (5)

MyPyramid. A personalized food system that helps you plan a healthier diet. (4)

N

National Adoption Information Clearinghouse. A national agency that offers adoption information to the public. (2)

needs. Items and services you must have in order to survive. (3)

net pay. Amount of your paycheck after taxes and deductions are taken out; also called take-home pay. (3)

networking. Talking with others to learn about job opportunities and openings. (7)

no-fault divorce. Type of divorce in which the partners do not have to prove grounds for divorce. (2)

noncustodial parent. Parent who does not reside with the children; nonresidential parent. (2)

nonresidential parent. Parent who does not reside with the children; noncustodial parent. (2)

Nutrition Facts label. Label that appears on almost all food products to provide nutritional information about the product. (4)

O

occasional expenses. Costs that arise from time-to-time rather than on a regular basis. (3)

occupational training. A training course or program that prepares a person to do work in a certain career field. (6)

order of protection. Court order that sets specific terms to protect a person or family from domestic violence that has been occurring. (2)

overdrawing. The act of writing checks, making purchases, or withdrawing money your account cannot cover. (5)

P

paternity. Biological fatherhood of a child; can be voluntarily admitted or proven through testing. (2)

paternity suit. Court case in which a child's mother sues the man she claims is the child's father; requests the court to order a paternity test. (2)

paternity test. Test done to prove whether a man is a child's biological father; can be a blood test or tissue test. (2)

payday loan. Money loaned against future paychecks; also called a cash-advance, check-advance, or delayed-deposit loan. (6)

payee. Person or company to whom a check or money order is written. (5)

personal identification number (PIN). Number, known by only you and the bank, that identifies your account and lets you use an ATM card or debit card to make transactions involving your account. (5)

physical custody. Type of custody that involves living with a child and providing physical care. (2)

post-dated check. Check dated for a given time in the future. (5)

premium. The fee you must pay for insurance. (5)

preventative care. Medical care that seeks to prevent problems or lessen their effect with early detection and treatment. (5)

probationary period. Time during which you, as a new employee, are evaluated on the work you do and how well you fit into the workplace. (7)

R

reference. A person who knows you well and is willing to speak to potential employers on your behalf. (7)

referral. A suggestion given by a professional of other services you might need. (1)

registered apprenticeship. An advanced apprenticeship program that requires a high school diploma or GED. (6)

regular charge account. Sales credit account that lets you charge your purchases and pay them in full when you receive a statement. (5)

release form. Form signed by the birthparents to allow someone else to take their baby from the hospital after birth. (2)

renter's insurance. Type of insurance coverage that protects the possessions of people who rent their homes. (5)

repossess. To take back an item purchased on credit; done by a creditor when the account is not repaid as agreed. (5)

residential parent. Parent with whom a child resides; custodial parent. (2)

resources. Any and all tools you can use to help you reach your goals. (3)

restrictive endorsement. Type of endorsement that tells what is to be done with a check; includes signature, account number, and directions for the bank. (5)

resume. Document that tells an employer what you have to offer as an employee. (7)

revolving credit account. Sales credit account that lets you charge purchases to a stated dollar limit and carry a balance from month-to-month. (5)

routine expenses. Expenses that must be paid on a regular basis. (3)

S

sales credit. Type of credit that lets you buy goods and services using a credit card or charge account. (5)

savings account. Bank account where you can keep your money safe for future use and possibly earn interest income on it. (5)

scholarship. A special award that pays all or part of college tuition and other costs. (6)

school-to-work program. Work-based learning program that prepares students for the workplace. (6)

search engine. Tool that searches the World Wide Web for specific information. (1)

seasonal sales. Sales put on by a store at the same time each year to get rid of seasonal items. (4)

Section 8 housing. Another name for subsidized housing. (1)

secured loan. Loan that requires some sort of security, such as collateral, a cosigner, or both. (5)

self-control. The ability to monitor your own actions and make appropriate choices. (4)

short-term goals. Goals that must be met within a few months. (3)

signature card. Bank card on which you give your official signature; the only signature the bank will honor on your financial transactions. (5)

single payment loan. Cash credit loan in which you repay the entire loan in one payment at a set time in the future. (5)

soft skills. Skills that will help you manage your life so you can hold a full-time job. (6)

sole custody. Custody arrangement in which only one parent has physical and legal custody of the children. (2)

special endorsement. Type of endorsement used to transfer to someone else a check that is written to you; includes signature, account number, and directions for the bank. (5)

Special Supplemental Nutrition Program for Women, Infants, and Children (WIC). Federal aid program that gives food vouchers, nutrition counseling, and medical screening to women who are pregnant or breast-feeding and their young children. (1)

States Children's Health Insurance Program (SCHIP). A national program that helps insure children who do not have insurance. (1)

subsidized housing. Low-income housing option in which the government pays part of a person's rent or mortgage, and he or she is responsible for the rest; sometimes called Section 8 housing. (1)

T

Temporary Assistance for Needy Families (TANF) Bureau. Federal aid bureau that includes cash assistance; replaced Aid to Families with Dependent Children (AFDC). (1)

term insurance. Type of life insurance policy that pays death benefits while the policy is in force but does not build cash value. (5)

U

unit price. The price of an item per unit, weight, or measure; used to compare cost across different sizes and brands of a product. (4)

unsecured loan. Loan made on a person's strong credit rating alone; requires no security. (5)

U.S. Department of Health and Human Services. Department of the federal government that focuses on meeting the health and service needs of the public. (1)

V

Vaccines for Children Program (VFC). Aid program that provides free immunizations for qualifying children. (1)

visitation rights. Court-approved rights of a nonresidential parent to see his or her children. (2)

W

wage withholding order. Court order that is sent to a person's employer and requires the employer to withhold part of the employee's wages and send them to the court; often done with child support payments. (2)

wants. Items and services you would like to have but can live without. (3)

warranty. Guarantee (often in writing) from a product maker that the product is well made and the company intends to stand behind it. (4)

WIC. See Special Supplemental Nutrition Program for Women, Infants, and Children (WIC). (1)

will. Legal document that states how a person wants his or her affairs managed after he or she dies. (2)

withdraw. To remove money from your checking or savings account. (5)

work ethic. A standard of conduct and values for job performance. (6)

work-study program. Program offered by many colleges in which students are connected with jobs on campus. (6)

Y

youth apprenticeship. An apprenticeship program designed for high school students. (6)

Index